Case-Based Discussions in Medicine

Dedication

To my patients and teachers, without whom this book would not be possible.

For Charlene, Isla, Emily and Freya. You are, as always, my inspiration!

Case-Based Discussions in Medicine

Paul James McNamara BSc (Hons) MBChB

Registrar in Emergency Medicine, Royal Hospital for Children, Glasgow

Honorary Clinical Lecturer, University of Glasgow School of Medicine

Scion

© **Scion Publishing Ltd, 2020**

First published 2020

A CIP catalogue record for this book is available from the British Library.

ISBN 9781911510482

Scion Publishing Limited

The Old Hayloft, Vantage Business Park, Bloxham Road, Banbury OX16 9UX, UK

www.scionpublishing.com

Important Note from the Publisher

The information contained within this book was obtained by Scion Publishing Ltd from sources believed by us to be reliable. However, while every effort has been made to ensure its accuracy, no responsibility for loss or injury whatsoever occasioned to any person acting or refraining from action as a result of information contained herein can be accepted by the authors or publishers.

Readers are reminded that medicine is a constantly evolving science and while the authors and publishers have ensured that all dosages, applications and practices are based on current indications, there may be specific practices which differ between communities. You should always follow the guidelines laid down by the manufacturers of specific products and the relevant authorities in the country in which you are practising.

Although every effort has been made to ensure that all owners of copyright material have been acknowledged in this publication, we would be pleased to acknowledge in subsequent reprints or editions any omissions brought to our attention.

Registered names, trademarks, etc. used in this book, even when not marked as such, are not to be considered unprotected by law.

Our medical textbooks are assessed and reviewed by the following medical students:

Nora Al Jamil	Sophie Gunter	Macauley Shaw
Tanith Bain	Laura Hartley	Aayushi Singal
Susan Baird	Zoe Johnson	Jay Singh
Nabeela Bhaloo	Victoria Kinkaid	Tanya Ta
Amy Campbell	Dylan McClurg	Bhavesh Tailor
Thomas Charles	Connor McKee	Paris Tatt-Smith
Yasmine Cherfi	Kate McMurrugh	Jack Whiting
Amaan Din	Marco Narajos	
Umar Dinah	Ross Porter	

We are grateful for their essential feedback. If you would like to apply to be a student reviewer, please contact **simon.watkins@scionpublishing.com** in the first instance.

Typeset by Medlar Publishing Solutions Pvt Ltd, India
Printed in the UK

Last digit is the print number: 10 9 8 7 6 5 4 3 2 1

Contents

Chapter 3: Obstetrics, gynaecology and paediatrics 145

Chapter 4: Psychiatry 187

Appendix: Figure acknowledgements *221*

Preface

Case-based learning (CBL) is now a fundamental approach to teaching medical students: 'The goal of CBL is to prepare students for clinical practice, through the use of authentic clinical cases'.

This book is a study companion for medical students and foundation doctors. It takes the reader through core clinical cases and aims to help the user become proficient at writing up a patient's history and examination findings.

During medical school, we are told that the patient's history and examination is our most valuable diagnostic tool. As students on the wards, you will have sufficient time to take comprehensive histories and examinations as they are presented in this book. Upon qualification, you will tailor your skills and the information the patient gives you to allow a more focused history and examination.

The cases presented will help to improve clinical decision-making, clinical knowledge and patient management.

Using real-life patient histories, each clinical presentation is followed by a commentary on the condition relating specifically to the presenting problem. Patients are presented as encountered 'on the job' and cases conclude with a discussion in terms of anatomy, physiology and pathophysiology,

thus giving a true reflection of disease processes and how they commonly present. Current guidelines, scoring systems and other classification criteria are also included.

A wide range of common presentations are covered. Each allows the reader to follow the patient's journey. Each case covers a number of areas, including:

▶ history-taking

▶ record-keeping

▶ clinical findings and interpretation

▶ management plan

▶ follow-up and future planning.

Taken together, the cases will give confidence in dealing with common medical and surgical conditions and emergencies. Medicine is a rapidly evolving field, so please note that this book is intended to be used with current guidelines.

As Mahatma Gandhi said, 'the best way to find yourself is to lose yourself in the service of others.' It is hoped that this book will guide you to medical success and help you to gain the competencies required to become confident and knowledgeable doctors.

Paul McNamara

About the author

Dr Paul McNamara is a registrar in emergency medicine. He graduated with a first-class honours degree in Anatomy.

He studied medicine at Glasgow University and qualified with a distinction and commendation. In medical school, Paul received numerous awards from the British Medical Association, The Cross Trust and The Trades House of Glasgow for academic achievement.

Paul has a keen interest in research and teaching. In 2017, he was awarded honorary clinical lecturer by the University of Glasgow for his contribution to teaching. He has published articles in the *British Medical Journal* and abstracts in the *Scottish Medical Journal* and *Clinical Anatomy*. He is a mentor for the Reach Foundation, which encourages school students from disadvantaged backgrounds to consider tertiary education and gives them access to medical work experience.

Abbreviations

AA	Alcoholics Anonymous
AAA	abdominal aortic aneurysm
ABCDE	Airway; Breathing; Circulation; Disability; Exposure
ABG	arterial blood gas
ACE	angiotensin-converting enzyme
ADH	antidiuretic hormone
AF	atrial fibrillation
AFP	alpha-fetoprotein
ALD	alcoholic liver disease
alk phos	alkaline phosphatase
ALT	alanine transaminase
AMA	anti-mitochondria antibody
ANA	anti-cell nuclei antibody
APER	abdomino-perineal resection
ASMA	anti-smooth muscle antibody
AST	aspartate transaminase
AV	atrioventricular
AVM	arteriovenous malformation
AVPU	alert, verbal, pain, unresponsive
AXR	abdominal X-ray
BCG	Bacillus Calmette–Guérin
bd	*bis in die* (twice daily)
BMI	body mass index
BP	blood pressure
bpm	beats per minute
CA-125	cancer antigen 125
CBL	case-based learning
CBT	cognitive behavioural therapy
CIN	cervical intraepithelial neoplasia
CNS	central nervous system
CO	cardiac output
COPD	chronic obstructive pulmonary disease
COX	cyclooxygenase
CRP	C-reactive protein
CT	computed tomography
CVA	cerebrovascular accident
CXR	chest X-ray
DVT	deep venous thrombosis
ECG	electrocardiography
ECT	electroconvulsive therapy
EPSE	extrapyramidal side-effect
ERCP	endoscopic retrograde cholangiopancreatography
ERPC	evacuation of retained products of conception
ESR	erythrocyte sedimentation rate
FAP	familial adenomatous polyposis
FBC	full blood count
FEV_1	forced expiratory volume in 1 second
FIGO	International Federation of Gynecology and Obstetrics

FVC	forced vital capacity
GABA	gamma-aminobutyric acid
gamma-GT	gamma-glutamyltransferase
GFR	glomerular filtration rate
GI	gastrointestinal
GORD	gastro-oesophageal reflux disease
GP	general practitioner
GTN	glyceryl trinitrate
Hb	haemoglobin
HbA1c	glycated haemoglobin
hCG	human chorionic gonadotrophin
HDL	high-density lipoprotein
HDU	high-dependency unit
HFE	hereditary haemochromatosis gene
HLA	human leukocyte antigen
HMG CoA-reductase	3-hydroxy-3-methyl-glutaryl-coenzyme A reductase
HNPCC	hereditary non-polyposis colorectal cancer
HPV	human papillomavirus
HR	heart rate
IBS	irritable bowel syndrome
IgE	immunoglobulin E
IL	interleukin
INR	international normalised ratio
ITU	intensive treatment unit
IV	intravenous
IVU	intravenous urogram
JVP	jugular venous pulse
KUB	kidney, ureters and bladder
LFT	liver function test
LIF	left iliac fossa
LKM	liver kidney microsome antibody
LLETZ	large loop excision of the transformation zone
LMP	last menstrual period
LOC	loss of consciousness
LV	left ventricular
LVEF	left ventricular ejection fraction
LVF	left ventricular failure
LVSD	left ventricular systolic dysfunction
mane	morning
MCV	mean corpuscular volume
MDT	multidisciplinary team
MI	myocardial infarction
MRI	magnetic resonance imaging
MS	multiple sclerosis
NAFLD	non-alcoholic fatty liver disease
NBM	nil by mouth
NG	nasogastric
NKDA	no known drug allergies
NMDA	*N*-methyl-D-aspartic acid
NOAC	new oral anticoagulant
nocte	night
NSAID	non-steroidal anti-inflammatory drug
NSCLC	non-small cell lung cancer
O_2 sats	oxygen saturation
OCSP	Oxfordshire Community Stroke Project
od	*omni die* (once daily)
PAF	platelet-activating factor
PCI	percutaneous coronary intervention
PEFR	peak expiratory flow rate
PID	pelvic inflammatory disease
PND	paroxysmal nocturnal dyspnoea
PO	*per os* (by mouth)
PPI	proton pump inhibitor
PR	*per rectum* (rectal)
prn	*pro re nata* (as needed)
PTH	parathyroid hormone
PV	*per vagina* (vaginal)
PVD	peripheral vascular disease
RBBB	right bundle branch block

RIF	right iliac fossa	tds	*ter die sumendus* (three times daily)
RR	respiratory rate	TFTs	thyroid function tests
RV	right ventricular	TIA	transient ischaemic attack
SAH	subarachnoid haemorrhage	TNF-alpha	tumour necrosis factor alpha
SaO$_2$	arterial oxygen saturation	TNM	tumour – nodes – metastases
SBR	serum bilirubin level	TSH	thyroid-stimulating hormone
SCLC	small cell lung cancer	TURBT	transurethral resection of bladder tumour
SOB	shortness of breath	U+Es	urea and electrolytes
SSRI	selective serotonin reuptake inhibitor	UC	ulcerative colitis
STEMI	ST elevation MI	UTI	urinary tract infection
TACS	total anterior circulation stroke	WCC	white cell count
TB	tuberculosis		
TCC	transitional cell carcinoma		

Chapter 1:

Medicine

Case 1: Progressive dyspnoea

Presenting complaint

▶ JL is an 84-year-old man who presented to hospital with a three-month history of progressive dyspnoea and fatigue.

History of presenting complaint

▶ JL first became symptomatic 1 year ago. He is a rather poor historian but remembers being very fatigued and had noticed that his ankles had begun to swell.

▶ JL also describes progressive-onset exertional dyspnoea. The shortness of breath (SOB) had been going on for several months, but has been getting progressively more frequent recently. In the past, it occurred with strenuous activity. Now it occurs with minimal exertion.

▶ Three months ago, JL was unable to walk 50 yards without feeling breathless, and he was having difficulty with activities of daily living such as climbing the stairs, washing and dressing.

▶ JL had an echocardiogram 3 weeks ago. On his way home, JL collapsed whilst walking and briefly lost consciousness on his driveway. JL has a very poor memory of the events that followed and is unaware of how he got to hospital.

▶ His breathlessness was not associated with any chest pain or palpitations. He does, however, report a persistent productive cough consisting of white sputum over the past 2–3 months, and he has orthopnoea and occasional paroxysmal nocturnal dyspnoea.

Past medical history

▶ Urticaria (2004)
▶ Myocardial infarction (1993)
▶ Duodenal ulcer
▶ Hernia repair
▶ No known history of diabetes or hypertension.

Drug history

Drug	Class	Dose	Frequency	Indication
Candesartan	Angiotensin-II receptor antagonist	4 mg	od	Heart failure
Bumetanide	Loop diuretic	2 mg	od	Pulmonary oedema due to left ventricular failure
Cetirizine	Non-sedating antihistamine	10 mg	od	Urticaria

Drug	Class	Dose	Frequency	Indication
Omeprazole	Proton pump inhibitor	20 mg	od	Duodenal ulcer
Aspirin	COX inhibitor	75 mg	od	Cardioprotection
Spironolactone	Aldosterone antagonist	100 mg	od	Heart failure
Bendroflumethiazide	Thiazide diuretic	5 mg	od	Oedema

Allergies

▸ No known drug allergies (NKDA).

Family history

▸ Father died aged 70 from oesophageal cancer.

▸ Mother died aged 76 from 'leg ulcers and cardiac asthma'.

▸ JL has a sister who also suffers from 'swollen legs'.

Social history

▸ JL has been married to his wife for 49 years; she experiences respiratory symptoms.

▸ They have one son (43 years old) and one daughter (47 years old). He says both are well.

▸ He has four grandchildren and two great-grandchildren.

▸ JL and his wife live in a terraced house. Since the onset of oedema in his legs, he has had significant problems with mobility. He has difficulty climbing the stairs despite handrails being fitted.

▸ JL worked as a labourer for 40 years.

▸ His social support consists of his wife and children.

▸ JL drank heavily in the past. When questioned further about this he was unwilling to elaborate, simply saying that he 'drank too much'.

▸ He now seldom drinks alcohol.

▸ He is an ex-smoker, having quit in 1994. He smoked 40 cigarettes/day for 40 years (80 pack-years).

Systemic enquiry

▸ **Neurological:** occasional headaches, poor vision, hearing aid in right ear. No dizziness, faints or seizures. No weakness or paraesthesia.

- **Cardiovascular:** breathlessness at rest, orthopnoea and occasional paroxysmal nocturnal dyspnoea (PND). No palpitations. Gross oedema of the legs to above the knee.

- **Respiratory:** persistent irritating productive cough (white sputum). JL says that he is 'exhausted' by it. No wheeze or haemoptysis.

- **Genitourinary:** nil.

- **Gastrointestinal:** chronic dyspepsia. No abdominal pain. One episode of melaena 2 weeks ago which he attributes to an episode of constipation. No overall change in bowel habit. No nausea or vomiting.

- **Musculoskeletal:** generalised muscle cramps, especially in the hands and legs. No pain or weakness in any joint.

Physical examination

General

- Elderly, slightly overweight man who is sitting upright and is clearly breathless. He is cyanosed and has a pale complexion.

Vital signs

- Temperature 36.4°C

- Blood pressure (BP) 105/50 mmHg

- Heart rate (HR) 60 bpm (beats per minute), regular

- Respiratory rate (RR) 22 breaths/minute

- Arterial oxygen saturation (SaO_2) 95%.

Neurological

- Patient is orientated to person, time and place

- Motor: good bulk and tone; strength is 5/5 throughout

- Cerebellar: finger–nose, heel–shin and rapid alternating movement responses are intact.

Cardiovascular

- No visible jugular venous pulse (JVP)

- Unable to palpate apex beat

- S1, S2; regular rate; no murmurs

- Bilateral leg oedema to level above the knee

- Unable to palpate posterior tibial and dorsalis pedis pulses, probably due to severity of bilateral leg oedema rather than peripheral vascular disease (PVD).

> **❶ Top tip**
>
> *How you would tell the difference between PVD and pedal oedema?*
>
> The most reliable physical findings of PVD are diminished or absent pedal pulses, presence of femoral artery bruit, abnormal skin colour, and cool skin temperature. JL had none of these. His main clinical sign was gross pedal oedema.

Respiratory

▶ No use of accessory muscles

▶ Tachypnoea

▶ Thorax symmetrical with good expansion

▶ Right lung resonant; vesicular breath sounds

▶ Left basal mid-inspiratory crackles

▶ Dyspnoeic at rest.

Gastrointestinal/abdominal

▶ No spider naevi or signs of anaemia; no hepatic flap

▶ Inguinal hernia scar

▶ Hepatomegaly

▶ Distended, non-tender abdomen.

Musculoskeletal

▶ Full range of movement in all joints; no deformities.

⚑ Red flags

▶ Unprovoked exertional collapse

▶ Dyspnoea at rest, orthopnoea and PND.

☰ Summary of patient's problems

▶ Dyspnoea at rest

▶ Bilateral leg oedema to above the knee

▶ Poor mobility related to dyspnoea and fatigue.

❓ Questions

▶ Based on the patient's symptoms, what are the main differential diagnoses?

▶ What initial investigations would help confirm the diagnosis?

▶ What is your immediate management plan?

Differential diagnosis

History and examination make left ventricular systolic failure the most likely diagnosis. JL had bilateral crepitations in his chest and gross pedal pitting oedema.

Consider what further investigations would rule out the other potential differential diagnoses below:

▶ pneumonia (productive purulent sputum, fever, consolidation on chest X-ray [CXR])

▶ bronchiectasis (chronic condition, does not normally present acutely – productive cough, frequent exacerbations, stereotypical computed tomography [CT] findings)

▶ fibrosis (dyspnoea, usually no peripheral oedema, or PND)

▶ asthma/chronic obstructive pulmonary disease (COPD) (possible but again not normally associated with pedal oedema)

▶ lung cancer (usually a history of chest discomfort, weight loss, haemoptysis)

▶ chronic renal failure (can cause oedema, but more unlikely given JL's other symptoms).

Management plan

▶ Oxygen (100%)

▶ Gain IV access

▶ Bloods – full blood count (FBC), urea and electrolytes (U+Es), C-reactive protein (CRP), troponins, brain natriuretic peptide (BNP)

▶ Electrocardiography (ECG) – look for signs of myocardial infarction (MI)

▶ CXR – look for cardiomegaly, signs of pulmonary oedema: shadowing, small effusions at costophrenic angles, fluid in the lung fissures, and Kerley B lines (linear opacities)

▶ Echocardiogram – can indicate cause of heart failure and may indicate left ventricular (LV) dysfunction

▶ Morphine 5 mg IV

▶ Furosemide 40–80 mg IV

▶ Leg ultrasound to exclude deep venous thrombosis (DVT).

Results of investigations

Chest X-ray

Pulmonary oedema and cardiomegaly: look for shadowing, small effusions at costophrenic angles, fluid in the lung fissures, and Kerley B lines (linear opacities).

Leg ultrasound

The femoral and popliteal veins compress fully and show normal augmented flow on calf compression, with no signs of femoropopliteal DVT in either leg.

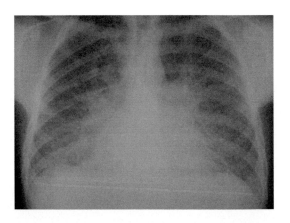

ECG

‣ Sinus rhythm

‣ Right bundle branch block (RBBB).

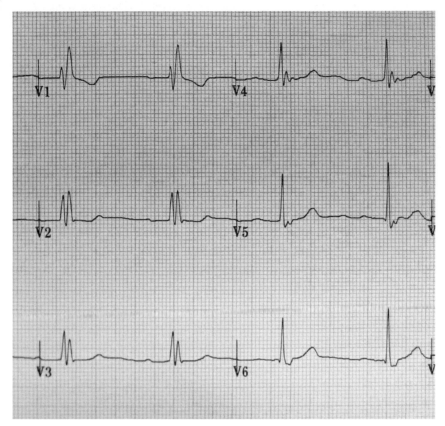

Characteristic changes in RBBB: delayed activation of the right ventricle results in an rsR pattern in V1 and a wide negative S wave in V6 (mnemonic MaRRoW).

Echo

Severe left ventricular systolic dysfunction (LVSD).

❓ Question

‣ What pharmacological treatments should be considered for the long-term management of heart failure?

Diagnosis

▸ Pulmonary oedema secondary to LVSD.

The combination of dyspnoea, PND and orthopnoea coupled with the examination findings such as crepitations in JL's chest and bilateral pedal oedema strongly suggest LVSD.

The diagnosis is made by the CXR findings of cardiomegaly and pulmonary oedema. His echo also confirmed severe LVSD.

Further management plan

▸ Daily weighing; BP and pulse/6 h

▸ Repeat CXR

▸ Change to oral furosemide or bumetanide

▸ Angiotensin-converting enzyme (ACE) inhibitor for LVF (left ventricular failure)

▸ Beta-blocker and spironolactone

▸ Consider digoxin (if atrial fibrillation [AF])

Background information: heart failure

Heart failure is defined as the inability of the heart to pump blood forward at a sufficient rate to meet the metabolic demands of the body (forward failure), or the ability to do so only if the cardiac filling pressures are abnormally high (backward failure) or both. Prognosis is very poor, with 82% of patients dying within 6 years of diagnosis.

Epidemiology

Approximately 920 000 people in the UK have heart failure. Both the incidence and prevalence of heart failure increase with age, with the average age of diagnosis being 77 years (NICE NG106, 2018).

Aetiology

Chronic cardiac failure can result from any structural or functional cardiac disorder that impairs the ability of the heart to function as a pump to support circulation. Causes of heart failure include:

▸ ischaemic heart disease (the most common cause in Western countries)

▸ (dilated) cardiomyopathy

▸ hypertension

▸ (undilated) cardiomyopathy

▸ valvular disease

▸ congenital heart disease

▸ alcohol and drugs, e.g. chemotherapy

▸ hyperdynamic circulation

▸ right heart failure (RV infarct, pulmonary hypertension, pulmonary embolism, cor pulmonale (COPD))

▸ arrhythmias (AF, bradycardia)

▸ pericardial disease.

The aetiologies of heart failure can be classified into three groups:

▸ impaired ventricular contractility

▸ increased afterload

▸ impaired ventricular filling.

Systolic dysfunction results from an abnormality of ventricular emptying (due to impaired contractility or excessive afterload), whereas diastolic dysfunction is caused by abnormalities of diastolic relaxation or ventricular filling.

LVF and right ventricular failure may occur independently, or may co-exist as congestive heart failure.

Pathophysiology

Several compensatory mechanisms are seen in patients with heart failure. These mechanisms buffer the fall in cardiac output and initially act to improve BP. They include:

▸ the Frank–Starling mechanism

▸ neurohormonal mechanisms

▸ the development of ventricular hypertrophy and remodelling.

Frank–Starling mechanism

Heart failure caused by left ventricular contractile dysfunction leads to decreased stroke volume. This results in incomplete chamber emptying, so more blood than normal accumulates in the ventricle. This increased stretch on the myofibres, acting through the Frank–Starling mechanism, induces a greater stroke volume on subsequent contraction, and helps to maintain cardiac output (CO). However, the effect is limited. Marked depression of cardiac contractility, as occurs in heart failure, is associated with elevated end-diastolic volume and pressures, and fluid accumulation is transmitted retrograde to the atrium, pulmonary veins and capillaries, and may result in pulmonary congestion and oedema.

Neurohormonal mechanisms

These include alterations in:

▸ the adrenergic nervous system

▸ the renin–angiotensin–aldosterone system

▸ production of antidiuretic hormone (ADH) – increases.

These mechanisms increase systemic vascular resistance, increase HR and improve contractility, increase circulating volume and ultimately help to perfuse vital organs. However, the beneficial effects are short-lived. Circulating volume is increased via the renin–angiotensin–aldosterone system and raised production of ADH, but it worsens the engorgement of the lungs and increases SOB. Furthermore, the elevated systemic vascular resistance increases the afterload against which the failing heart has to contract and further impairs stroke volume and hence CO. The increased HR increases the metabolic demands of the myocardium and negatively affects its function. In addition, chronic stimulation of the adrenergic nervous system leads to down-regulation of receptors and a reduced inotropic response. It is also known that continually elevated levels of angiotensin II and aldosterone cause fibrosis and adverse remodelling of the heart.

Symptoms and signs

The symptoms depend on which ventricle is more affected:

Left ventricular failure	Right ventricular failure
Dyspnoea, poor exercise tolerance, fatigue, orthopnoea, PND, nocturnal cough (+/– pink frothy cough), wheeze, nocturia, cold peripheries, weight loss, muscle wasting.	Peripheral oedema, ascites, nausea, anorexia, facial engorgement, pulsation in neck and face, epistaxis.

Signs include:

▶ general: looks ill and exhausted, cool peripheries, peripheral cyanosis

▶ pulse: resting tachycardia, pulsus alternans

▶ BP: low, narrow pulse pressure, raised JVP*

▶ praecordium: displaced apex* (LV dilatation), RV heave (pulmonary hypertension)

▶ auscultation: S3 gallop*, murmurs of aortic or mitral disease

▶ chest: tachypnoea, bi-basal end-inspiratory crackles*, wheeze, pleural effusions

▶ abdomen: hepatomegaly, ascites, peripheral oedema*

*Signs most specific for congestive cardiac failure.

Heart failure can be classified depending on severity as shown in the table below.

New York Heart Association classification	
I	No limitation: ordinary physical exercise does not cause undue fatigue, dyspnoea or palpitations
II	Slight limitation of physical activity: comfortable at rest but ordinary activity results in fatigue, palpitations or dyspnoea
III	Marked limitation of physical activity: comfortable at rest but less than ordinary activity results in symptoms
IV	Unable to carry out any physical activity without discomfort: symptoms of heart failure are present even at rest with increased discomfort with any physical activity

Pharmacological therapy

Treatment according to SIGN (147, 2016) and NICE guidelines (NG106, 2018) is intended to prevent progression, thereby reducing symptoms, hospital admissions and mortality.

Diuretics

Diuretics are a key element of heart failure treatment. Diuretic therapy is associated with a reduction in oedema and breathlessness. A loop diuretic is usually used, e.g. furosemide 40 mg/24 h PO.

ACE inhibitors

Studies (CONSENSUS, SOLVD) have shown that ACE inhibitors such as enalapril and captopril are associated with decreased mortality and reduced hospitalisations in people with heart failure.

JL was not receiving an ACE inhibitor. However, he is known to have chronic renal failure, which may explain this deviation from the guidelines, or he may have had an adverse effect such as cough. He is, however, taking candesartan (4 mg), which is in line with current recommendations.

Beta-blockers

Beta-blockers such as carvedilol have been shown (BEST [Beta-blocker Evaluation of Survival Trial], CIBIS-II [Cardiac Insufficiency Bisoprolol Trial II], COPERNICUS [Carvedilol Prospective Randomized Cumulative Survival Study], and MERIT-HF [Metoprolol Randomized Intervention Trial in Congestive Heart Failure] to decrease mortality in people with heart failure. One should be administered on a 'start low, go slow' policy with regular assessment of BP and pulse.

Spironolactone

The RALES trial showed that spironolactone (25 mg/24 h PO) reduced mortality by 30%

when added to conventional therapy and is therefore recommended for use in people with heart failure.

Digoxin

Digoxin should be considered as an add-on therapy in people with deteriorating symptoms despite optimum therapy. Dose: 0.125–0.25 mg/24 h.

Resources

European Society of Cardiology *Clinical Practice Guidelines: Acute and Chronic Heart Failure* (2016): www.escardio.org/Guidelines/Clinical-Practice-Guidelines/Acute-and-Chronic-Heart-Failure

NICE *Chronic heart failure in adults: diagnosis and management: Guideline 106* (2018): www.nice.org.uk/guidance/ng106

SIGN *Management of chronic heart failure, Guideline 147* (2016): www.sign.ac.uk/sign-147-management-of-chronic-heart-failure.html

Case 2: Wheeze

Presenting complaint

▶ MG is a 54-year-old female smoker with chronic asthma who presented with wheeze, dyspnoea and a productive cough.

History of presenting complaint

▶ MG presented to her GP two weeks ago with exertional dyspnoea and wheeze. She also had a productive cough (green sputum).

▶ She had no chest pain, haemoptysis or fever.

▶ The GP prescribed a course of steroids and amoxicillin.

▶ However, this had little effect on her symptoms and she returned to her GP yesterday. Examination by the GP revealed that she was tachycardic (HR 150 bpm), had widespread wheeze, and was hypoxic (oxygen saturation [O_2 sats] 95%).

▶ Her peak expiratory flow rate (PEFR) was unrecordable.

▶ While receiving oxygen at the GP surgery, she became dizzy and unwell and O_2 sats dropped to 85%. She was subsequently transferred by ambulance to the acute medical unit (AMU).

Past medical history

▶ Chronic asthma (diagnosed 1989). Usually well controlled. No previous admissions.

▶ No diabetes or hypertension.

Drug history

Drug	Class	Dose	Frequency	Indication
Salbutamol (Ventolin)	Beta agonist	200 mcg	prn	Asthma
Tiotropium (Spiriva)	Antimuscarinic bronchodilator	18 mcg	od	Asthma
Fluticasone propionate (in Seretide)	Corticosteroid	100 mcg	od	Asthma prophylaxis

Allergies

▶ NKDA.

Family history

- Her father died at the age of 47 from 'heart problems'.

- Mother passed away at 66 from an MI.

- She has two younger sisters and a younger brother. Her brother has an arrhythmia and one of her sisters has had an MI.

- No family history of asthma.

Social history

- MG has been married to her husband for 35 years. They live in a 3-bed semi-detached house with their 25-year-old son.

- She works as a customer service adviser for BT.

- She has smoked 20 cigarettes per day for 30 years (30 pack-years). She is a social drinker.

Systemic enquiry

- **Neurological:** No falls, loss of consciousness (LOC), seizures or dizziness. Occasional headaches.

- **Cardiovascular:** No ankle oedema or chest pain.

- **Respiratory:** SOB; no PND or orthopnoea. Wheeze. Productive cough.

- **Genitourinary:** No dysuria, frequency, history of urinary tract infection (UTI) or nocturia.

- **Gastrointestinal:** No change in bowel habit. No melaena. No abdominal pain or nausea and vomiting. Poor appetite.

- **Musculoskeletal:** No pain or stiffness in any joint.

Physical examination

General

- MG talks in sentences but is clearly breathless.

- She is warm and well perfused.

- No pallor, jaundice, cyanosis or clubbing.

Vital signs

- BP 152/92 mmHg
- HR 129 bpm – regular
- RR 20 breaths/minute
- O_2 sats 93% on air.

Cardiovascular

▸ No visible JVP

▸ Apex beat in fifth intercostal space in the mid-clavicular line

▸ S1, S2; regular rate

▸ Peripheral pulses present

▸ No oedema.

Respiratory

▸ No use of accessory muscles

▸ Tachypnoea

▸ Thorax symmetrical; poor expansion

▸ Dyspnoeic at rest

▸ Widespread bilateral wheeze; prolonged expiratory phase.

☰ Summary of patient's problems

▸ Dyspnoea at rest

▸ Hypoxia

▸ Productive cough and wheeze

▸ Difficulty completing sentences.

❷ Questions

▸ Based on the patient's symptoms, what are the main differential diagnoses?

▸ What initial investigations would help confirm the diagnosis?

▸ What is your immediate management plan?

Differential diagnosis

▶ Asthma

▶ Foreign body obstruction – may cause a localised wheeze depending on site; no significant improvement on bronchodilators

▶ Cardiac dysfunction – is there a history of LV dysfunction with signs and symptoms of heart failure including crackles on auscultation of the lungs and peripheral oedema?

▶ Anaphylaxis – more stridor than wheezing. Is there a history of exposure to stimulus?

▶ Emphysema/COPD – COPD exacerbations and asthma exacerbations are clinically similar, with cough, SOB, and wheezing

▶ Pneumothorax – can present with symptoms similar to an asthma exacerbation; SOB and chest tightness are common symptoms.

Management plan

▶ ABCDE approach (Airway; Breathing; Circulation; Disability; Exposure)

▶ Salbutamol 5 mg plus ipratropium bromide 0.5 mg nebulised with oxygen

▶ Prednisolone 40 mg PO (consider IV hydrocortisone if vomiting or gastric absorption impaired)

▶ Gain IV access

▶ Bloods including FBC, U+Es, CRP, liver function tests (LFTs), blood cultures if pyrexial

▶ CXR – look for pneumothorax/consolidation

▶ ECG

▶ Arterial blood gas (ABG)

▶ DVT prophylaxis

▶ Monitor PEFR and O_2.

❷ Question

▶ What other treatments might be considered if she fails to improve?

Results of investigations

Blood results

Substance	Reference range	Result
Na$^+$	135–145 mmol/L	138 mmol/L
Cl$^-$	96–105 mmol/L	103 mmol/L
ALT	<50 U/L	80 U/L

(continued overleaf)

Substance	Reference range	Result
Alk phos	30–130 U/L	47
Gamma-GT	F <32 U/L, M <50 U/L	211 U/L
Bilirubin	<20 µmol/L	6 µmol/L
CRP	<1 mg/L	2 mg/L
Hb	135–155 g/L	115 g/L
Ca^{2+}	2.12–2.65 mmol/L	2.18 mmol/L
MCV	76–96 fL	109.2 fL
WCC	$4–11 \times 10^9$/L	13×10^9/L
Neutrophils	40–75%	6%
Platelets	$150–400 \times 10^9$/L	282×10^9/L
ESR		6 mm/hour

Na^+, sodium ions; Cl^-, chloride ions; ALT, alanine transaminase; alk phos, alkaline phosphatase; gamma-GT, gamma-glutamyltransferase; CRP, C-reactive protein; Hb, haemoglobin; Ca^{2+}, calcium ions; MCV, mean corpuscular volume; WCC, white cell count; ESR, erythrocyte sedimentation rate.

ECG

Sinus tachycardia; normal axis.

CXR

Hyperinflation.

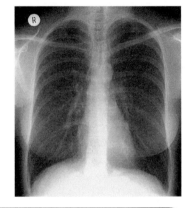

PEFR

▸ Normally 250–300 L/min

▸ Before nebuliser 100 L/min

▸ After nebuliser 140 L/min.

Diagnosis

▸ Acute exacerbation of asthma

The combination of dyspnoea, wheeze and productive cough coupled with the examination findings of low O_2 sats and reduced PEFR strongly suggest a diagnosis of acute exacerbation of asthma.

Further management plan

If life-threatening features are observed, add magnesium sulphate 1.2–2.0 g IV over 20 minutes and then either IV aminophylline **or** IV salbutamol (or terbutaline).

Consider transfer to intensive treatment unit (ITU) for mechanical ventilation if no improvement.

Background information: asthma

Asthma is characterised by chronic airway inflammation and increased airway hyper-responsiveness leading to symptoms of wheeze, cough, chest tightness and dyspnoea. It is functionally characterised by airflow obstruction that is variable over short periods of time, or is reversible with treatment. The prevalence of asthma has been increasing steadily over the past few decades. In childhood it is more common in boys, but following puberty women are more frequently affected.

Aetiology and pathogenesis

The aetiology of asthma is complicated. The recent increase in incidence has been linked to the 'hygiene hypothesis' – decreased exposure to infection in early childhood is believed to bias the immune system towards an allergic phenotype. Asthma is also found among atopic individuals and families. Atopy is an inherited predisposition to sensitisation to allergens. Atopic individuals have an increased risk of allergic disease such as eczema, allergic rhinitis and asthma. Asthmatics may also have a genetic predisposition to airway hyper-responsiveness.

Asthma is characterised by:

▶ airflow limitation (usually reversible spontaneously or with treatment)

▶ hyper-responsiveness of the airway to a wide range of stimuli

▶ inflammation of bronchi with T lymphocytes, mast cells, eosinophils with associated plasma exudation, oedema, smooth muscle hypertrophy, matrix deposition, mucus plugging and epithelial damage.

Investigations

There is no single diagnostic test for asthma. A CXR should be performed to exclude other causes at first presentation. In asthma, the CXR may show hyperinflation (due to air trapping) and areas of collapse (due to mucus plugging).

In preschool children, assessment is largely clinical. Older children and adults should be encouraged to perform PEFR measurements. Measurements on waking, before taking a bronchodilator and before bed are particularly useful in demonstrating the variable airflow limitation that characterises asthma. Spirometry may also be performed. Skin-prick testing or measuring specific immuno-globulin E (IgE) to various allergens may be helpful in identifying important allergies that could be targets for exposure reduction.

Treatment

The aims of asthma treatment are:

▶ achieve and maintain the control of symptoms

▶ prevent exacerbations

▶ maintain pulmonary function as close to normal as possible

▶ avoid adverse effects from asthma medication

▶ prevent the development of irreversible airflow limitation

▶ prevent asthma mortality.

The treatment of asthma consists of a stepwise approach in accordance with the SIGN/BTS guidance (2016). Patients may be placed at the bottom (step 1) of the plan or a higher step if their symptoms warrant stronger medication. The stepwise approach allows patients to step down or step up their medication according to their condition.

STEP 5 – Continuous frequent use of oral steroids (lowest dose possible for adequate control)

STEP 4 – Persistent poor control
▸ Increase inhaled steroid to high/max dose
▸ Add 4th line drug, e.g. leukotriene receptor antagonist, β_2-agonist tablets, SR theophylline

STEP 3 – Poorly controlled on inhaled steroids
▸ Add inhaled long-acting β_2-agonist, e.g. salmeterol
▸ Assess response: good response – continue
inadequate benefit– increase inhaled steroid

STEP 2 – Requires ≥ 3 β_2-agonist inhalations per week
▸ Add inhaled corticosteroid, e.g. beclometasone

STEP 1 – Mild intermittent asthma
▸ Inhaled short-acting β_2-agonist as required, e.g. salbutamol
▸ Consider ipratropium bromide in infants/young children

Based on BTS/SIGN 2016 guidelines.

Management of acute severe asthma

Severe attack:

▸ Unable to complete sentences

▸ RR > 25/min (23 on admission)

▸ HR >110 bpm (104 on admission)

▸ PEFR < 50% of predicted or best.

Life-threatening attack:

▸ PEFR < 33% of predicted or best

▸ Silent chest, cyanosis, weak respiratory effort

▸ Bradycardia or hypotension

▸ Exhaustion, confusion or coma

▸ ABG: normal/high PCO_2 > 4.6 kPa
PO_2 < 8 kPa or O_2 sats < 92%.

❓ Question

▸ What severity of asthma attack is MG having?

Start treatment immediately (before investigations):

▸ Sit patient up and give high-flow oxygen

▸ Salbutamol 5 mg plus ipratropium bromide nebulised with O_2

▸ Hydrocortisone 100 mg IV or prednisolone 40–50 mg PO

▸ CXR to exclude pneumothorax.

If the patient is improving, oxygen and frequency of nebulisers can be reduced with monitoring of PEFR and O_2 sats. However, if the patient does not improve after 15–30 minutes, continue with high-flow oxygen and steroids, and increase the frequency of salbutamol nebulisers to every 15 minutes.

If the attack has life-threatening features, add magnesium sulphate 1.2–2.0 g IV over 20 minutes and then either IV aminophylline **or** IV salbutamol (or terbutaline).

Consider transfer to ITU for mechanical ventilation if no improvement.

Resources

BTS/SIGN *British guideline on the management of asthma, Guideline 153* (2016 – due for update late 2019): www.sign.ac.uk/sign-153-british-guideline-on-the-management-of-asthma.html or www.brit-thoracic.org.uk/quality-improvement/guidelines/asthma/

Case 3: Chest pain

Presenting complaint

▶ AR is a 61-year-old man who presented with acute chest pain.

History of presenting complaint

▶ AR developed sudden-onset central chest pain whilst at rest. The pain was dull in nature and did not radiate. The pain was accompanied by breathlessness and sweating, but no nausea or vomiting.

▶ He describes the pain as constant and severe, and he was frightened by the experience. He was not aware of any palpitations.

Past medical history

▶ Ulcerative colitis   ▶ Pulmonary fibrosis

▶ No known history of angina, diabetes, hypertension or hyperlipidaemia.

Drug history

▶ Before admission: prednisolone 15 mg od and alfacalcidol.

Allergies

▶ NKDA.

Family history

▶ Mother died aged 87 ('old age')

▶ Father died aged 80 ('old age')

▶ 4 brothers and 1 sister

▶ No known family history of cardiovascular disease.

Social history

▶ AR lives alone in a one-bedroom flat. He has no children.

▶ He has worked as an electrician for 46 years, but has been unable to work for the last 6 months due to pulmonary fibrosis.

- He has never smoked.
- He is a heavy drinker and admits to drinking 5–6 pints/night.

Systemic enquiry

- **Neurological:** No dizziness, faints or seizures. No muscle weakness or paraesthesia.
- **Cardiovascular:** Severe chest pain. No palpitations. Exertional dyspnoea. No paroxysmal nocturnal dyspnoea or orthopnoea. No ankle swelling.
- **Respiratory:** SOB. No cough and wheeze. No haemoptysis.
- **Genitourinary:** Nil.
- **Gastrointestinal:** No dyspepsia. No abdominal pain or change in bowel habit.
- **Musculoskeletal:** Nil.

Physical examination

General

- Distressed gentleman. Grey complexion and sweating profusely. Obviously breathless.

Vital signs

- BP 125/91 mmHg
- RR 14 breaths/minute
- HR 70 bpm – irregularly irregular
- O_2 sats 97% on air.

Cardiovascular

- No visible JVP
- Apex beat in fifth intercostal space in the mid-clavicular line
- S1, S2; irregular rate
- Peripheral pulses present
- No oedema.

Respiratory

- No clubbing or CO_2 flap
- Trachea is central and no lymphadenopathy
- Equal chest expansion
- Fine inspiratory crackles in both lung fields.

Summary of patient's problems

▸ Severe chest pain at rest

▸ SOB

▸ Autonomic activation (sweating profusely).

Questions

▸ Based on the patient's symptoms, what are the main differential diagnoses?

▸ What initial investigations would help confirm the diagnosis?

▸ What is your immediate management plan?

Differential diagnosis

- Acute coronary syndrome
- Pulmonary embolism
- Pneumonia/pleurisy
- Musculoskeletal chest pain
- Pneumothorax

Management plan

- Assess ABCDE
- Oxygen (100%)
- IV access and analgesia (morphine 5 mg IV + metoclopramide 10 mg IV)
- Nitrate (GTN) and 300 mg aspirin (chewed)
- Bloods (FBC, U+Es, CRP, troponins)
- ECG – look for signs of MI
- CXR – look for cardiomegaly, signs of pulmonary oedema: shadowing, small effusions at costophrenic angles, fluid in the lung fissures, and Kerley B lines (linear opacities)
- Echocardiogram (in due course).

Results of investigations

Blood results

Substance	Reference range	Result
Na$^+$	135–145 mmol/L	137 mmol/L
ALT	<50 U/L	32 U/L
AST	<40 U/L	112 U/L
Gamma-GT	F <32 U/L, M <50 U/L	71 U/L
Bilirubin	<20 µmol/L	16 µmol/L
Hb	135–155 g/L	139 g/L
MCV	76–96 fL	91 fL
WCC	4–11 × 10^9/L	8.8 × 10^9/L
Neutrophils	40–75%	4.8%
Platelets	150–400 × 10^9/L	363 × 10^9/L
Glucose		4.8 mmol/L
Troponin*	F <16 ng/L, M <34 ng/L	2225 ng/L
Cholesterol	5 mmol/L	5.50 mmol/L

Na$^+$, sodium ions; ALT, alanine transaminase; AST, aspartate transaminase; gamma-GT, gamma-glutamyltransferase; Hb, haemoglobin; MCV, mean corpuscular volume; WCC, white cell count.

*Troponin levels will vary depending on regional labs. However, note markedly elevated troponin.

ECG

Acute anterior ST elevation myocardial infarction (STEMI).

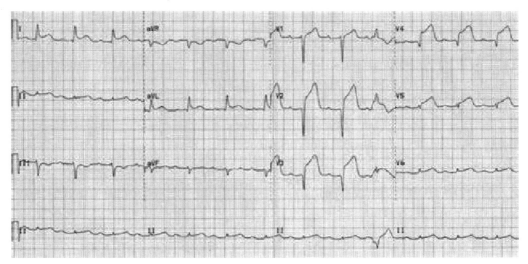

Diagnosis

▶ Acute anterior STEMI

This patient presented with sudden-onset central chest pain whilst at rest. The pain did not radiate but it was associated with pallor, profuse sweating and dyspnoea. Combined with the positive troponin and stereotypical ECG findings, this confirmed the diagnosis. After the diagnosis of acute anterior STEMI, the patient developed AF.

❓ Question

▶ What are the treatment options now?

Background information: STEMI

STEMI is caused by thrombus formation on a ruptured atheromatous plaque in the coronary arteries. Treatment aims to restore coronary blood flow, either via primary percutaneous coronary intervention (PCI) or thrombolytic therapy.

PCI is an invasive procedure using balloon angioplasty and stents to open the blocked artery. It is superior to thrombolysis but it is limited by its availability at specialist centres only.

Primary PCI is recommended as the treatment of choice, if the patient can receive treatment within 90 minutes. If this is not possible, then the patient should receive thrombolytic therapy. Given that the ECG changes were consistent with STEMI and AR lived close to a national cardiac centre, he was transferred for PCI.

The alternative of thrombolytic therapy involves the use of drugs such as tenecteplase to break up the clot in the coronary arteries. There is a risk of bleeding. Contraindications include previous stroke, gastrointestinal (GI) bleeding, recent surgery and bleeding disorders.

Secondary prevention

▶ **Aspirin:** maintenance dose 75 mg; antiplatelet drug; prevents re-infarction.

▶ **Ticagrelor:** maintenance dose 90 mg; antiplatelet drug; prevents re-infarction post-MI, in addition to aspirin – prescribed for 6 months.

▶ **Statin:** simvastatin 40 mg; cholesterol-lowering drug (an HMG-CoA reductase inhibitor).

▶ **Beta-blocker:** bisoprolol 2.5 mg initially (increasing up to 10 mg if tolerated); cardioselective beta-blocker.

▶ **ACE inhibitor:** ramipril 2.5 mg. Shown to reduce mortality post-MI; greatest benefit in patients with left ventricular dysfunction and heart failure.

> **❷ Question**
>
> ▶ What complications can occur with acute myocardial infarction?

Complications of acute MI:

▶ **atrial arrhythmia** – the most common is AF

▶ ventricular arrhythmia

▶ bradycardia

▶ heart failure

▶ cardiogenic shock

▶ myocardial rupture

▶ pericarditis

▶ LV mural thrombus.

AR's post-MI progress was complicated by AF.

Atrial tachyarrhythmias arise from the atrial myocardium and include AF, atrial flutter atrial tachycardia and atrial ectopic beats.

Background information: AF

AF is a chaotic, irregular rhythm with an atrial rate so fast that discrete P waves are not discernible on the ECG. The atrioventricular (AV) node responds intermittently, producing an irregular ventricular rate. AF may be paroxysmal (lasting <48 hours) or permanent.

Epidemiology

AF is a common arrhythmia, occurring in 5–10% of over-65s. The paroxysmal form is more common in younger patients.

Aetiology

Any condition that results in raised atrial pressure, increased atrial muscle mass, atrial fibrosis or inflammation and infiltration of the atrium may cause AF.

Cardiac factors in AF	Non-cardiac factors in AF
Hypertension	Thyrotoxicosis
Congestive heart failure	Phaeochromocytoma
Coronary heart disease and MI	Acute and chronic pulmonary disease (pneumonia, COPD)
Valvular heart disease	Pulmonary vascular disease (pulmonary embolism)
Cardiomyopathy (dilated, hypertrophic)	Electrolyte disturbance (hypokalaemia)
Myocarditis and pericarditis	Alcohol abuse ('holiday heart', long-term use)
Wolff–Parkinson–White syndrome	Caffeine, smoking, recreational drug use
Sick sinus syndrome	
Cardiac tumours	
Cardiac surgery	
Familial tachyarrhythmia (e.g. lone AF)	

Pathophysiology

AF is thought to be the result of multiple meandering re-entry wavelets driven by rapidly depolarising autonomic foci. The atria respond electrically to this rate, but there is no co-ordinated mechanical action and only a proportion of the impulses are conducted to the ventricles. Because the ventricles are not reliably primed by the atria, the cardiac output drops by 10–20%. Furthermore, the absence of organised atrial contraction promotes blood stasis, leading to an increased risk of thrombus formation. Embolisation of left atrial thrombi is an important cause of stroke.

Symptoms

▸ Asymptomatic (30%)

▸ Chest pain

▸ Palpitations

▸ Dyspnoea

▸ Faintness

▸ Deterioration of exercise capacity.

Signs

▸ Irregularly irregular pulse

▸ Signs of LVF: distressed, pale, sweaty, tachycardia, tachypnoea, frothy pink sputum, pulsus alternans, increased JVP, fine lung crackles

▸ Signs of systemic disease

Investigations

▸ ECG – absent P waves, irregular QRS complexes

▸ Bloods – Hb (?anaemia), U+Es, cardiac enzymes, thyroid function tests (TFTs)

▸ CXR – look for signs of LVF

▸ Echo – look for left atrial enlargement, mitral valve disease, poor LV function and other structural abnormalities.

Treatment

The most important thing about treating AF is to treat the patient, not the ECG. One must consider how well the arrhythmia is tolerated (signs of decompensation include chest pain, hypotension, pulmonary congestion, decreased level of consciousness) and whether spontaneous cardioversion is likely.

If AF is found to be due to an acute precipitating event (e.g. alcohol toxicity, chest infection, hyperthyroidism) the provoking cause should be treated.

The aims of treating AF include:

▸ restoration of sinus rhythm

▸ rate control

▸ anticoagulation assessment.

Restoration of sinus rhythm

Cardioversion (electronic or medical) may be considered in individuals who are likely to return to and stay in sinus rhythm (first episode of AF, young) or in the acutely unwell. Electrical DC cardioversion 200 J, then 2 × 360 J achieves sinus rhythm in ~80% of patients. Anticoagulation is used to minimise the risk of thromboembolism associated with cardioversion unless the duration of AF is <48 hours. Patients must be anticoagulated with warfarin or NOAC for 4 weeks or have a transoesophageal echo to determine the presence or absence of atrial thrombus.

Medical cardioversion is possible with an intravenous infusion of an antiarrhythmic drug such as class Ic (flecainide 2 mg/kg over >25 minutes) or class III agents (amiodarone 5 mg/kg over 1 hour, then 900 mg over 24 hours via a central line – risk of thrombophlebitis) if there is structural heart disease. Flecainide is a sodium-channel blocker that reduces myocardial excitability. Class III antiarrhythmic drugs are potassium-channel blockers. Amiodarone also blocks sodium and calcium channels to prolong the cardiac action potential duration and prolong the effective refractory period. Or, if a particular drug has been shown to be safe in a particular patient, an oral agent may be administered ('pill in the pocket' approach).

Rate control in AF

Rate control should be considered when the patient is >65 years old. Coronary artery disease, contraindications to antiarrhythmics and contraindications to cardioversion are also indications for rate control as opposed to rhythm control. Rate control can be achieved by class II (β-blockers) and class IV agents (calcium antagonists: verapamil and diltiazem) and digoxin. Beta-blockers and calcium channel blockers promote block at the AV node and reduce ventricular rate. They should not be given together. Digoxin is not included in the Vaughan Williams classification of antiarrhythmics. It is a cardiac glycoside which slows AV conductance and shortens the atrial action potential by stimulating vagal activity. In addition, digoxin is a positive inotrope, so is useful in patients, like AR, with accompanying impairment of ventricular contractile function.

Anticoagulation

Heparin should be used in acute AF until a full risk assessment for emboli is made. The CHA_2DS_2-VASc score can be used to assess the need for long-term anticoagulation therapy.

CHA_2DS_2-VASc score

Abbreviation	Risk factor	Points
C	Congestive heart failure (LVEF <40%)	1
H	Hypertension	1
A	Age ≥75 years	2
D	Diabetes mellitus	1
S	Stroke/TIA or systemic embolism	2
V	Vascular disease	1
A	Age 65–74 years	1
Sc	Sex category (female)	1

LVEF, left ventricular ejection fraction; TIA, transient ischaemic attack.

Long-term anticoagulation is with the vitamin K antagonist warfarin (target international normalised ratio [INR] 2–3) or new oral anticoagulant (NOAC) e.g. apixaban.

Contraindications to warfarin	
Absolute contraindications	**Relative contraindications**
Potential bleeding lesions Active peptic ulcer, oesophageal varices, aneurysm, proliferative retinopathy	History of GI bleed Liver disease Renal failure Alcoholism

(continued overleaf)

Contraindications to warfarin *(continued)*	
Absolute contraindications	**Relative contraindications**
Recent organ biopsy	Mental impairment
Recent trauma or surgery to head, orbit or spine	Thrombocytopenia
	Coagulation disorders
Recent stroke	
Confirmed intracranial or intraspinal bleed	Interacting drugs, e.g. NSAIDs
	Frequent falls
Uncontrolled hypertension	Poor attendance for regular blood tests
Infective endocarditis	

NSAID, non-steroidal anti-inflammatory drug.

Warfarin is metabolised by the cytochrome P450 system. Therefore many drugs can interact with its metabolism and hence its effect.

Drugs that interact with warfarin	
Cytochrome P450 inhibitors (increase the effect of warfarin)	**Cytochrome P450 inducers (decrease the effect of warfarin)**
Antibiotics (erythromycin, ciprofloxacin, metronidazole, co-trimoxazole, isoniazid)	Antiepileptics (carbamazepine, phenytoin)
	Rifampicin
Antifungals (fluconazole)	Chronic alcohol consumption
Cimetidine	Barbiturates
Omeprazole	Sulphonylureas
Sodium valproate	
Acute alcohol consumption (binge drinking)	

Resources

European Society of Cardiology *Clinical Practice Guidelines: Atrial fibrillation* (2016) www.escardio.org/Guidelines/Clinical-Practice-Guidelines/Atrial-Fibrillation-Management

European Society of Cardiology *Clinical Practice Guidelines: Acute myocardial infarction in patients presenting with ST-segment elevation* (2017): www.escardio.org/Guidelines/Clinical-Practice-Guidelines/Acute-Myocardial-Infarction-in-patients-presenting-with-ST-segment-elevation-Ma

NICE *Atrial fibrillation: Clinical guideline 180* (2014): www.nice.org.uk/guidance/cg180

NICE *Myocardial infarction with ST-segment elevation: acute management: Clinical guideline 167* (2013): www.nice.org.uk/guidance/cg167

NICE guidance: www.nice.org.uk/guidance/conditions-and-diseases/cardiovascular-conditions/acute-coronary-syndromes

SIGN *Acute coronary syndrome, Guideline 148* (2016): www.sign.ac.uk/sign-148-acute-coronary-syndrome.html

Case 4: Dyspnoea and confusion

👤 Presenting complaint

▸ MG is a 36-year-old lady with known COPD who presented with increased breathlessness and confusion.

History of presenting complaint

▸ On the day of admission, MG was found at home confused, disorientated and extremely breathless. She has a history of COPD, and when her mother checked her O_2 saturations she was only saturating at 73% on air.

▸ She was subsequently admitted to hospital and was treated for an acute exacerbation of COPD.

▸ She says that she had no cough, fever, chest pain or haemoptysis. However, while on the ward, MG woke up with a dense right-sided weakness affecting the arm and leg and causing marked right-sided facial droop. There was no visual disturbance, reduced consciousness, or loss of bowel or bladder control.

Past medical history

▸ MG was diagnosed with α-1-antitrypsin deficiency 3 years ago. She feels that her symptoms are now static and she uses domiciliary oxygen, which helps.

▸ There is no known history of diabetes, hypertension, epilepsy, MI or stroke.

Drug history

Drug	Dose	Frequency	Indication
Seretide	1 puff	bd	COPD
Omeprazole	20 mg	od	GORD
Tiotropium	18 mcg	od	COPD
Salbutamol nebuliser	2.5 mg	od	COPD
Carbocisteine (mucolytic)	750 mg	tds	COPD
Prednisolone	40 mg	od – 4 days	COPD

Allergies

▸ Penicillin

Family history

▸ Nil

Social history

▸ She lives with her parents and 7-year-old daughter in a 2-bedroom flat.

▸ She says that she is independent, but is inhibited somewhat by the two flights of stairs leading up to her flat. This stops her from leaving the home and she is resigned to the fact that she will need home help.

▸ She has never worked.

▸ She is a non-smoker and non-drinker.

Systemic enquiry

▸ **Neurological:** No dizziness, faints or seizures. Right-sided hemiplegia and dysphasia.

▸ **Cardiovascular:** No chest pain or palpitations. Breathlessness at rest. No paroxysmal nocturnal dyspnoea or orthopnoea.

▸ **Respiratory:** SOB. Productive cough and wheeze. No haemoptysis.

▸ **Genitourinary:** Nil.

▸ **Gastrointestinal:** No dyspepsia. No abdominal pain or change in bowel habit.

▸ **Musculoskeletal:** Nil.

Physical examination

General

▸ MG is a lady who looks older than her age, sitting comfortably upright and in no obvious pain or discomfort.

▸ She appears pale, breathless at rest and is centrally cyanosed. On nasal O_2. Inhalers and O_2 tank by the bed.

Vital signs

▸ BP 110/60 mmHg

▸ HR 99 bpm – regular

▸ RR 20 breaths/minute

▸ O_2 sats 96% on 3 L.

Neurological

	Right leg	Right arm	Left leg	Left arm
Power	2/5	2/5	5/5	5/5
Tone	Normal	Normal	–	–
Reflexes	Increased	Increased	–	–

Cardiovascular

▶ No visible JVP

▶ Apex beat in fifth intercostal space in the mid-clavicular line

▶ S1, S2; regular rate

▶ Peripheral pulses present

▶ No oedema.

Respiratory

▶ No clubbing or CO_2 flap

▶ Trachea is central and no lymphadenopathy

▶ Tachypnoea

▶ Reduced chest expansion

▶ Bilateral basal crepitations and widespread wheeze.

☰ Summary of patient's problems

▶ Dyspnoea at rest   ▶ Acute confusion and disorientation

▶ Hypoxia   ▶ Acute dense right-sided weakness.

❷ Questions

▶ Based on the patient's symptoms, what are the main differential diagnoses?

▶ What initial investigations would help confirm the diagnosis?

▶ What is your immediate management plan?

Differential diagnosis

Right-sided hemiparesis and dysphasia:

▸ Cerebrovascular accident (CVA) (most likely)

▸ Central nervous system (CNS) tumour

▸ Cerebral abscess

▸ Trauma – subdural haematoma, traumatic brain injury

▸ Multiple sclerosis (MS)

▸ Todd's palsy – limb weakness following a seizure: the patient seems to have had a stroke, but recovers in 24 hours

▸ Migraine

▸ Hypoglycaemia.

Management plan

▸ Assess ABCDE**FG** (never **f**orget **g**lucose!)

▸ Oxygen (cautious in COPD)

▸ Gain IV access

▸ Bloods – Hb (look for anaemia, polycythaemia), WCC (look for sepsis)

▸ Blood sugar – **mandatory** to detect treatable hypoglycaemia

▸ ABG

▸ Imaging: computed tomography (CT) to exclude CVA, bleeding, tumour, abscess
CXR to detect tumours or relevant lung pathology; assess heart size
carotid Doppler – to detect significant stenosis
cardiac echo – if any suspicion of intracardiac thrombus
ECG to detect significant dysrhythmia

▸ Assessment of swallowing

▸ Check BP and look for source of emboli.

Results of investigations

ABG on 28% O_2

▸ H^+ 41.5 mmol/L

▸ PaO_2 6.9 kPa

▸ $PaCO_2$ 8.3 kPa

▸ HCO_3^- 36.7 mmol/L

▸ Lactate   0.4 mmol/L

▸ Base excess   9.6 mmol/L.

❓ **Question**

▸ What does the blood gas show?

The ABG measurement showed type 2 respiratory failure with a compensatory metabolic alkalosis.

CXR

The CXR showed evidence of hyperinflation but no focal changes consistent with acute infection.

ECG

Rate 85 bpm; sinus rhythm; right axis deviation; no acute changes.

CT brain

Hypoattenuation and loss of grey/white matter differentiation.

Diagnosis

▸ Acute cerebrovascular infarct

Two days after admission for COPD this patient developed a dense right-sided weakness, affecting the arm and leg and causing marked right-sided facial droop. A CT brain confirmed a hyperacute ischaemic stroke.

Further management plan

MG woke up with her hemiplegia. There was no definitive time of onset of her symptoms. She was therefore not commenced on thrombolysis. She was started on 300 mg aspirin.

❓ **Question**

▸ How would you classify this patient's stroke according to the Oxfordshire Community Stroke Project (OCSP) Classification?

Background information: stroke

Strokes can be either haemorrhagic or ischaemic. They are impossible to distinguish clinically and therefore imaging is essential.

The OCSP Classification is used to classify types of strokes.

MG had a left **total anterior circulation stroke (TACS)**. This is diagnosed when a stroke causes all three of the following symptoms:

▸ contralateral hemiparesis

▸ contralateral hemianopia

▸ higher dysfunction (e.g. dysphasia, visuo-spatial disturbances) +/– contralateral hemisensory loss.

Partial anterior circulation stroke (PACS) is diagnosed when two of the above three are present or when there is higher dysfunction alone e.g. isolated dysphasia.

Lacunar stroke (LACS) can present with:

▸ pure motor stroke/hemiparesis

▸ ataxic hemiparesis

▸ dysarthria/clumsy hand

▸ pure sensory stroke

▸ mixed sensorimotor stroke.

Posterior circulation stroke (POCS) can cause the following symptoms:

▸ cranial nerve palsy (ipsilateral) with contralateral motor/sensory defect

▸ bilateral motor or sensory defect

▸ eye movement disorder

▸ cerebellar signs

▸ isolated homonymous hemianopia.

Management plan

▸ Confirm clinical diagnosis

▸ Distinguish haemorrhagic/ischaemic stroke

▸ Look for underlying cause and direct therapy.

Consider:

▸ Long-term management

▸ Rehabilitation: physiotherapy and speech therapy.

Cerebral infarction

If CT shows infarction, give aspirin (300 mg/day initially) antiplatelet therapy if no contraindications, give alteplase thrombolysis, which must be started within 3 hours (aim for 90 minutes) of stroke; informed consent essential.

Cerebral haemorrhage

If CT shows haemorrhage, do not give any therapy that may interfere with clotting. Neurosurgery may be required.

Admit to multidisciplinary stroke unit if possible.

Background information: COPD

Chronic obstructive pulmonary disease (COPD) is not one single disease but an umbrella term used to describe chronic lung diseases that cause limitations in lung airflow. The airflow obstruction is the result of small airways disease (obstructive bronchitis) and alveolar destruction (emphysema), discrete pathological processes which make an independent contribution to the overall burden of airflow limitation in the affected individual.

Cigarette-smoking is the major environmental risk factor for the development of COPD. According to the WHO, 80 million people have moderate to severe COPD. It estimates that more than 3 million people died of COPD in 2005, which corresponds to 5% of all deaths globally.

The prevalence of COPD amongst women is on the increase due to the recent rise in the numbers of women who smoke. Total deaths from COPD are expected to increase if urgent action is not taken to reduce the underlying risk factors. Estimates suggest that by the year 2020 COPD will be the third leading cause of death globally.

Pathophysiology

COPD is an inflammatory disease with pulmonary and systemic effects. Physiologically it is characterised by airflow limitation, impaired gas exchange, hyperinflation and reduced efficiency of the respiratory muscles.

Pathological changes

Within the lungs COPD is associated with:

▶ an increase in the volume and number of submucosal glands

▶ an increase in the number of goblet cells in the mucosa

▶ mucosal inflammation

▶ emphysema

▶ loss of alveolar attachments to small airway

▶ inflammatory exudate within airway lumina.

Emphysema

Emphysema is defined as abnormal, permanent enlargement of airspaces distal to the terminal bronchiole, accompanied by destruction of their walls and without obvious fibrosis. Emphysema may be classified by the pattern of the enlarged airspaces: centriacinar, panacinar and periacinar. Bullae form in some individuals. This results in impaired gas exchange and respiratory failure.

Bronchitis

Chronic bronchitis is defined clinically as a daily cough with production of sputum for 3 months, 2 years in a row. Enlargement of mucus-secreting glands and an increase in the number of goblet cells, accompanied by an inflammatory cell infiltrate, results in an increase in sputum production leading to chronic bronchitis.

Clinical features

COPD should be suspected in any patient over the age of 40 years who presents with symptoms of persistent cough and sputum production and/or breathlessness. Cough is usually the first symptom and it is characteristically accompanied by small amounts of mucoid sputum. Breathlessness is usually the presenting complaint.

Grade	Degree of breathlessness related to activities
0	No breathlessness except with strenuous exercise
1	Breathlessness when hurrying on the level or walking up a slight hill
2	Walks more slowly than contemporaries on level ground because of breathlessness or has to stop for breath when walking at own pace
3	Stops for breath after walking about 100 m or after a few minutes on level ground
4	Too breathless to leave the house, or breathless when dressing or undressing

Exacerbations

Acute exacerbations of COPD are characterised by an increase in symptoms and deterioration in lung function and health status. An increase in the following symptoms is typical: dyspnoea, sputum purulence, sputum volume and cough. Acute exacerbations become more common as the disease progresses and may be caused by bacteria, viruses or a change in air quality. They may be accompanied by the development of respiratory failure and/or fluid retention, and are an important cause of death.

Bacteria are isolated from 40–60% of acute exacerbations of COPD. Three bacterial species account for most isolates: *Haemophilus influenzae*, *Streptococcus pneumoniae* and *Moraxella catarrhalis*.

Haemophilus influenzae is present in about 50% of culture-positive sputa in most clinical trials.

Diagnosis

COPD has an insidious onset and usually presents in the older population. A history of productive cough, wheezing and SOB, particularly with exercise, is typical. Patient's smoking history, occupational exposures and any family history of lung disease should be determined. Patients with COPD may also present with acute, severe SOB, fever and chest pain during acute infectious exacerbation.

Examination may show tachypnoea, respiratory distress, use of accessory muscles and intercostal retraction. Barrel chest is a common observation. There may be hyper-resonance on percussion, and distant breath sounds and poor air movement on auscultation. Wheezing, rhonchi, clubbing and cyanosis, as well as signs of right-side heart failure may be present.

Investigation

Spirometry is the first test for diagnosis of COPD and for monitoring disease progress. Patients with COPD have a distinctive pattern seen on spirometry with a reduced forced expiratory volume in 1 second (FEV_1) and FEV_1/FVC ratio (FVC: forced vital capacity). The presence of airflow limitation is defined by the GOLD criteria as a post-bronchodilator FEV_1/FVC less than 0.70. CXR is rarely diagnostic but can help to exclude other diagnoses. Pulse oximetry screens for hypoxia. Presence of purulent sputum is sufficient to commence empiric antibiotics in an acute exacerbation. If these fail, sputum should be sent for culture.

Treatment

COPD staging and therapy at each stage.

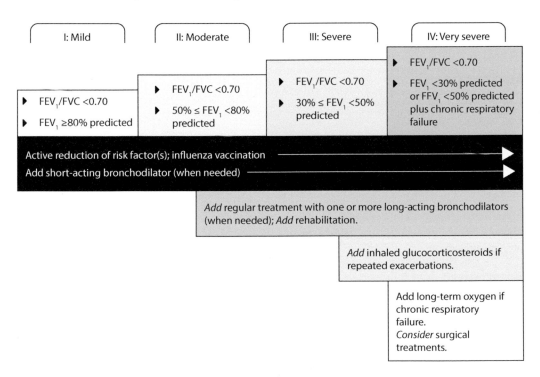

I: Mild	II: Moderate	III: Severe	IV: Very severe
▶ FEV_1/FVC <0.70 ▶ FEV_1 ≥80% predicted	▶ FEV_1/FVC <0.70 ▶ 50% ≤ FEV_1 <80% predicted	▶ FEV_1/FVC <0.70 ▶ 30% ≤ FEV_1 <50% predicted	▶ FEV_1/FVC <0.70 ▶ FEV_1 <30% predicted or FFV_1 <50% predicted plus chronic respiratory failure

Active reduction of risk factor(s); influenza vaccination
Add short-acting bronchodilator (when needed)

Add regular treatment with one or more long-acting bronchodilators (when needed); *Add* rehabilitation.

Add inhaled glucocorticosteroids if repeated exacerbations.

Add long-term oxygen if chronic respiratory failure.
Consider surgical treatments.

Ongoing monitoring and assessment in COPD ensures that the goals of treatment are being met. Such an assessment of the medical history should include:

Exposure to risk factors and preventative measures:

- Tobacco smoke

- Occupational exposures (fumes, dust, etc.)

- Influenza and pneumococcal vaccination.

Disease progression and development of complications:

- Decline in exercise tolerance

- Increased symptoms

- Worsened sleep quality

- Missed work or other activities.

Pharmacotherapy and other medical treatment:

- How often rescue inhaler is used

- Any new medicines

- Compliance with medical regimen

- Ability to use inhalers properly

- Side-effects.

Exacerbation history

- Urgent care or emergency department visits

- Recent oral corticosteroid bursts

- Frequency, severity and likely causes of exacerbations should be evaluated.

Comorbidities:

- Assessment of co-existing medical problems (e.g. heart failure).

In addition, objective assessment of lung function should be obtained yearly, or more frequently if there is a substantial increase in symptoms.

GOLD guidelines recommend a stepwise approach to therapy:

- For patients with stage I disease, short-acting bronchodilators are used first-line as required.

- In stage II disease, long-acting bronchodilators should be commenced in addition to as-required short-acting bronchodilators, and pulmonary rehabilitation is offered.

- In stage III disease, inhaled corticosteroid therapy is added to regular and as-required bronchodilators, if frequent exacerbations occur.

- Finally, in stage IV disease, long-term oxygen therapy should be added to inhaled therapies, and possible surgical interventions should be considered.

All patients are candidates for education, vaccination and smoking cessation interventions.

Background information: α-1-antitrypsin deficiency

Alpha-1-antitrypsin is a glycoprotein that belongs to a family of serine protease inhibitors involved in controlling inflammatory cascades. It is synthesised in the liver, and its deficiency is the chief genetic cause of liver disease in children. In adults, its lack causes emphysema.

Genetics

Alpha-1-antitrypsin deficiency is an autosomal recessive disorder. The gene is located on chromosome 14.

Pathophysiology

The genetic defect in α-1-antitrypsin deficiency alters the configuration of the α-1-antitrypsin molecule and prevents its release from hepatocytes. As a result, serum levels of α-1-antitrypsin are decreased, leading to low alveolar concentrations, where the α-1-antitrypsin molecule normally serves as protection against proteases. The resulting protease excess in alveoli destroys alveolar walls and causes emphysema.

The accumulation of excess α-1-antitrypsin in hepatocytes can also lead to destruction of these cells and, ultimately, clinical liver disease.

Investigations

▶ Serum α-1-antitrypsin levels are decreased

▶ Liver biopsy – periodic acid–Schiff (PAS) stain positive

▶ Phenotyping

▶ CT

▶ Lung function tests.

Management

Management is mostly supportive for emphysema and liver complications. Augmentation therapy with α-1-antitrypsin from human plasma can be considered if FEV_1 is less than 80% and the patient does not smoke; however, it is very expensive.

Resources

Global Initiative for Chronic Obstructive Lung Disease (GOLD): https://goldcopd.org/

Case 5: Back pain and breathlessness

👤 Presenting complaint

▶ MC is a 64-year-old gentleman who presented with low back pain and breathlessness.

History of presenting complaint

▶ MC has a 10-week history of pain in his lower back and right flank. The pain is constant and he describes it as a dull ache.

▶ Approximately 6 weeks ago, MC had a sudden onset of breathlessness. He is breathless at rest, but it is exacerbated by daily activities. He has no orthopnoea or PND.

▶ He also describes a pain in his chest and right shoulder. He is aware of a change in his voice and thinks that he is hoarse.

▶ There is no weight change, fever or night sweats. There is no cough but he does report an episode of dark sputum.

▶ He has been feeling more tired over the past few months.

Past medical history

▶ Dupuytren's contracture repair in both hands
▶ Chronic pain related to arthritis
▶ Spondylitis
▶ Anxiety/depression.

Drug history

Drug	Class	Dose	Frequency	Indication
Tramadol	Opioid	100 mg	4 hourly	Moderate to severe pain
Trazodone	Tricyclic related	100 mg	nocte	Depression
Temazepam	Benzodiazepine	10 mg	nocte	Anxiety
Gabapentin	GABA analogue	300 mg	1 tab	Neuropathic pain
Senna	Stimulant laxative	15 mg	2 tabs daily	Constipation
Lactulose	Semi-synthetic disaccharide	15 mL	×2	Constipation
Meloxicam	NSAID	15 mg	×2	Osteoarthritis
Valsartan	Angiotensin II receptor antagonist	80 mg	×2	Hypertension
Ranitidine	H_2-receptor antagonist	150 mg	mane	Gastric protection

Allergies

▸ NKDA.

Family history

▸ Mother died in her 60s from breast cancer

▸ Father died aged 82 from 'old age'.

Social history

▸ MC's wife died last year from breast cancer. This has understandably affected MC's psychological well-being and he says that he has been very depressed since his wife's death.

▸ He has a son who is 29 and a daughter who is 23.

▸ He lives in a 4-bedroom semi-detached house. Recently he has been finding it difficult to climb the stairs due to SOB.

▸ MC worked as a plasterer for 25 years.

▸ Drinks 8–14 units per week.

▸ Ex-smoker. Smoked 5/day for 16 years (4 pack-years). He quit 20 years ago.

Systemic enquiry

▸ **Neurological:** Two-week history of headaches ('burning'), central vision disturbance in right eye. No weakness or paraesthesia.

▸ **Cardiovascular:** Angina.

▸ **Respiratory:** Sudden onset SOB, initially on exertion, now at rest.

▸ **Genitourinary:** Nil.

▸ **Gastrointestinal:** Constipation. No abdominal pain or melaena.

▸ **Musculoskeletal:** Generalised pain. Osteoarthritis, spondylitis.

Physical examination

General

▸ MC is sitting in bed and is comfortable but appears slightly tachypnoeic.

Vital signs

▸ Temp 36.4°C

▸ HR 80 bpm, regular

▸ O_2 sats 95%.

▸ BP 125/70 mmHg

▸ RR 19 breaths/minute

Cardiovascular

▶ No visible JVP

▶ Apex beat palpable at the fifth interspace in the mid-clavicular line

▶ S1, S2; regular rate; no murmurs

▶ He is well perfused.

Respiratory

▶ No use of accessory muscles

▶ Tachypnoea

▶ Thorax symmetrical; poor expansion

▶ Scattered crepitations bilaterally

▶ Stony dull percussion on the left

▶ Dyspnoeic at rest.

Gastrointestinal/abdominal

▶ No spider naevi or signs of anaemia; no hepatic flap

▶ Soft and non-tender

▶ Bowel sounds present.

☰ Summary of patient's problems

▶ Deteriorating SOB

▶ Pain in his left shoulder and chest

▶ Hoarse voice.

---

❷ Questions

▶ Based on the patient's symptoms, what are the main differential diagnoses?

▶ What initial investigations would help confirm the diagnosis?

▶ What is your immediate management plan?

Differential diagnosis

▶ Lung cancer ▶ Pulmonary emboli

▶ TB ▶ Lower respiratory tract infection

▶ Pneumonia ▶ LVF.

Management plan

▶ Assess the patient using ABCDE

▶ Oxygen (100%)

▶ Gain IV access

▶ Pain relief – morphine 5 mg IV (titrate as required to patient response)

▶ Bloods (FBC, U+Es, CRP, troponins, D-dimers)

▶ CXR

▶ ECG.

Results of investigations

Blood results

Normal except markedly raised D-dimer
(4539: normal <230).

CXR

Left-sided pleural effusion

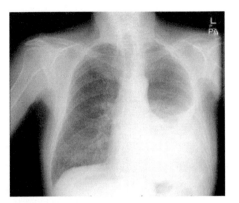

❷ Questions

▶ What is the most likely diagnosis now?

▶ What further investigations would help confirm the diagnosis?

Diagnosis

▶ Primary bronchial carcinoma

MC is an ex-smoker who complained of SOB and back pain. CXR was consistent with pleural effusion, and the most likely diagnosis is underlying bronchial carcinoma.

Further management plan

▶ Pleurocentesis microscopy result: pleural fluid contains abundant groups of malignant glandular epithelial cells; the immunohistochemical profile is in keeping with a pulmonary origin (EP4, CK7, TTF-1 positive).

▶ CT (staging)

▶ Multidisciplinary team (MDT) approach

▶ Continue with pain relief.

Background information: lung cancer

Lung cancer is the second most common cancer in Scotland after non-melanoma skin cancer. There are approximately 4800 new cases per year and 4000 deaths (SIGN 137, 2014). In the UK, bronchial carcinoma is the third most common cause of death after heart disease and pneumonia.

Aetiology

Smoking is the most common aetiological factor in lung cancer. Occupational factors include contact with asbestos, arsenic, chromium, iron oxides and the products of coal combustion.

Pathology

Bronchial carcinomas are broadly divided into small cell (SCLC) and non-small cell lung cancer (NSCLC).

Non-small cell lung cancer is further subdivided, depending on histology, into:

▸ squamous carcinoma (40%)

▸ adenocarcinoma (10%) – commonly associated with asbestos and non-smokers

▸ large cell carcinomas (25%)

▸ bronchoalveolar cell (1–2%) – presents as a peripheral solitary nodule or as diffuse nodular lesions of multicentric origin.

Clinical features

Local effects of the tumour within a bronchus may lead to common symptoms such as cough, chest pain, haemoptysis and breathlessness. Spread within the chest may involve the pleura and ribs, leading to pain and fractures. Involvement of the brachial plexus causes pain in the shoulder and inner arm (Pancoast tumour), whereas spread to the sympathetic ganglion causes Horner's syndrome, and spread to the left recurrent laryngeal nerve causes hoarseness and a bovine cough.

The tumour may also spread to the oesophagus, heart or superior vena cava and can cause upper-limb oedema, facial congestion and distended veins.

Patients may also present with features related to metastatic disease. Common sites of metastases include the bone, brain, liver and adrenals.

Lung cancer is also associated with extra-pulmonary manifestations such as:

▸ hypertrophic pulmonary osteoarthropathy – joint stiffness and severe pain in the wrist and ankles

▸ weight loss

▸ parathyroid hormone (PTH)-related peptide – hypercalcaemia

▸ clubbing

▸ syndrome of inappropriate secretion of ADH – dilutional hyponatraemia.

Management

According to guidelines (SIGN 137, 2014; NICE NG122, 2019), an urgent CXR should be offered to everyone presenting with haemoptysis, or any of the following if unexplained or lasting longer than 3 weeks:

▸ cough

▸ chest/shoulder pain

▸ dyspnoea

▸ weight loss

▸ chest signs

▸ hoarseness

▸ finger clubbing

▸ signs suggesting metastases

▸ cervical/supraclavicular lymphadenopathy.

Other relevant investigations include cytology (sputum/pleural fluid), percutaneous fine needle aspiration or biopsy, bronchoscopy and CT.

The treatment of lung cancer is dependent on the histological type and stage of disease. NSCLC is staged with the tumour – nodes – metastases (TNM) system, whereas SCLC is simply defined as extensive or limited, depending on spread.

The only treatment of any curative value for NSCLC is surgery with neo-adjuvant chemotherapy. Only 20% of cases are suitable for surgical resection. Of these, the 5-year survival rate is 25–30%. Lobectomy is the treatment of choice for those who can tolerate it. Radical radiotherapy treatment is also indicated in those with stage I, II and III NSCLC who have good performance status (based on WHO performance scale 0, 1).

In those who have stage III and IV disease, chemotherapy should be offered to improve survival and control the progress of the disease. Chemotherapy should be a combination of:

▶ a third-generation drug such as docetaxel, gemcitabine, paclitaxel or vinorelbine

▶ a platinum drug – carboplatin or cisplatin.

Chemotherapy in SCLC has resulted in a fivefold increase in median survival, from two months to five months. All patients should be offered multi-drug platinum-based chemotherapy. In those with limited disease, thoracic irradiation should be offered with the first or second cycle of chemotherapy. Chemotherapy should only be offered to patients with extensive disease if there has been a complete response to the chemotherapy at distant sites or at least a good partial response within the thorax.

Prognosis

After 2 years, 50% of patients with NSCLC are alive if there is no spread (10% if spread). The prognosis of SCLC is poor. The median survival is 3 months if untreated compared to 1–1.5 years if treated.

Resources

NICE *Lung cancer: diagnosis and management guideline NG122* (2019) www.nice.org.uk/guidance/ng122

SIGN *Management of lung cancer, Guideline 137* (2014): www.sign.ac.uk/sign-137-management-of-lung-cancer.html

Case 6: Headache

👤 Presenting complaint

▸ MM is a 35-year-old female who presented with an acute severe headache.

History of presenting complaint

▸ Five days ago, MM experienced a 'horrendous' headache. The headache occurred without warning and she says she felt like she had been 'hit on the back of the head'. The pain is described as sharp and localised to the right occipital region.

▸ The pain didn't radiate and was made worse by standing and moving around. It was associated with nausea but not vomiting. She has lost her appetite.

▸ She has not lost consciousness or had any seizures. The headache was not associated with weakness, paraesthesia, or visual disturbance.

▸ There is no neck stiffness or rash.

Past medical history

▸ Childhood asthma (last attack 7 years ago)

▸ Ovarian cyst.

Drug history

Drug	Class	Dose	Frequency	Indication
Ferrous fumarate	Oral iron	322 mg	od	Iron-deficiency anaemia (ovarian cyst)

Allergies

▸ NKDA.

Family history

▸ Mother died aged 54 years – ischaemic heart disease

▸ No other relevant family history.

Social history

▸ MM has been married for 11 years. She has a son (7) and a daughter (11).

- They live in a detached 3-bedroom house.
- She works as a district nurse.
- She drinks 10 units of alcohol/week and is a non-smoker.

Systemic enquiry

- **Neurological:** Acute severe headache. No photophobia, paraesthesia, weakness, neck stiffness. No visual, taste or hearing disturbances. No change in speech or swallowing.
- **Cardiovascular:** No chest pain, palpitations, or breathlessness.
- **Respiratory:** Nil.
- **Genitourinary:** Nil.
- **Gastrointestinal:** Nil.
- **Musculoskeletal:** Nil.

Physical examination

General

MM is lying in bed and appears unwell. She is pale and clammy but is easily roused.

Vital signs

- Temp 37.9°C
- HR 88 bpm
- BP 159/100 mmHg
- AVPU A
- RR 16 breaths/minute

Neurological

Inspection

- Good posture
- No muscle wasting or fasciculations; no abnormal movements such as tremor
- No arm drifting.

Tone

- Normal tone.

Power

- 5/5 throughout.

Reflexes

- Normal.

Cardiovascular

- No visible JVP
- Apex beat is palpable in the fifth interspace in the mid-clavicular line

- ▶ Heart sounds I + II; no murmurs
- ▶ Patient is rather pale, but is well perfused
- ▶ No oedema.

Respiratory

- ▶ Good chest expansion
- ▶ Good air-entry throughout; no added sounds.

Gastrointestinal/abdominal

- ▶ Abdomen is soft, slight tenderness in the left iliac fossa related to her ovarian cyst
- ▶ Bowel sounds present.

☰ Summary of patient's problems

- ▶ Sudden onset severe headache
- ▶ Nausea.

---

❷ Questions

- ▶ Based on the patient's symptoms, what are the main differential diagnoses?
- ▶ What initial investigations would help confirm the diagnosis?
- ▶ What is your immediate management plan?

Differential diagnosis

- Subarachnoid haemorrhage (SAH)
- Meningitis
- Migraine
- Viral encephalitis
- Sinusitis.

Management plan

- Assess the patient using ABCDE
- Pain relief – paracetamol (1 g/4 h) and diclofenac (50 mg/8 h)
- Reassess pain and modify pain relief according to WHO pain ladder; may require IV morphine
- Gain IV access
- Bloods – FBC, U+Es, LFTs, CRP, glucose, clotting, blood cultures
- ECG
- CT head.

Results of investigations

Blood results

- FBC normal
- LFT normal
- CRP < 5 mg/mL
- U+Es within normal range.

ECG

Normal.

CT head

Subarachnoid haemorrhage
(blood shows up as white).

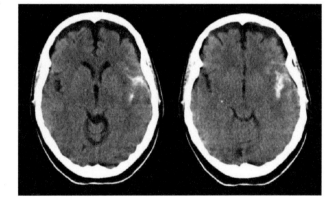

Diagnosis

- Subarachnoid haemorrhage

This patient presented with a 'thunderclap' occipital headache. This is strongly suggestive of SAH, and the diagnosis was confirmed on CT. If the CT had not shown any blood, the patient would have gone on to have a lumbar puncture.

Further management plan

- Continue analgesia and antiemetic
- Discuss with neurosurgeons.

Background information: SAH

Normal cerebral blood flow: the circle of Willis

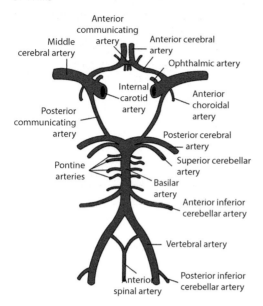

SAH means spontaneous rather than traumatic arterial bleeding into the subarachnoid space. SAH accounts for 5% of strokes and has an annual incidence of 6 per 100 000. The mean age of presentation is 50 years.

The underlying causes of SAH are:

▸ saccular ('berry') aneurysms – 70%

▸ arteriovenous malformation (AVM) – 10%

▸ no lesion identifiable – 20%.

The risk of subarachnoid haemorrhage is increased if the person smokes; excessively abuses alcohol; has hypertension; has a bleeding disorder; is a close relative of someone with SAH (3–5-fold increase in risk of SAH).

Saccular (berry) aneurysms

These develop on the circle of Willis and adjacent arteries. Common sites are:

▸ between the posterior communication and internal carotid artery (posterior communicating artery aneurysm)

▸ between anterior communicating and anterior cerebral artery (anterior communicating artery aneurysm)

▸ at the bifurcation of the middle cerebral artery (middle cerebral artery aneurysm).

Arteriovenous malformation (AVM)

AVM is an abnormal connection between arteries and veins within the brain that is of developmental origin. If an AVM ruptures, it has a tendency to rebleed, and 10% will then do so each year.

Clinical features

The symptoms caused by aneurysms are either the result of spontaneous rupture, where there is usually no preceding history, or by direct pressure on surrounding structures. In those that become symptomatic due to the mass effect, the most common symptom is painful third-nerve palsy. A lesion of the oculomotor nerve causes unilateral complete ptosis, the eye faces 'down and out', and the pupil is dilated and fixed to light and convergence.

The typical presentation of SAH is the sudden onset of severe headache. The pain is often localised to the occipital region, and it reaches maximum intensity immediately or after only minutes. It is often associated with nausea and vomiting, and sometimes loss of consciousness.

On examination there may be signs of meningeal irritation (neck stiffness and a positive Kernig's sign), focal neurological signs and subhyaloid haemorrhages (haemorrhages between the retina and vitreous membrane). Some patients may experience some minor headaches in the days leading up to the haemorrhage.

Differential diagnosis

Only 25% of sudden severe, 'thunderclap' headaches are due to subarachnoid haemorrhage. In the majority (50–60%), no cause is found. The remaining individuals have migraine, intracerebral bleeds, or cerebral venous thrombosis.

Investigations

The investigation of choice is CT. This should ideally be performed within 12 hours of symptoms. Lumbar puncture is only indicated if there is a strong clinical suspicion of an SAH but the CT scan is normal. An increase in bilirubin and/or oxyhaemoglobin (released from lysis and phagocytosis of red blood cells) is the key finding that indicates SAH. Furthermore, a magnetic resonance (MR) angiography is usually performed to identify the source of bleeding in all patients who are potentially fit for surgery.

Management

Immediate treatment consists of bed rest and supportive measures. Severe hypertension should be cautiously controlled. Dexamethasone may be prescribed to control cerebral oedema; it is also believed to stabilise the blood–brain barrier. Nimodipine, a calcium channel blocking agent, is given by mouth (60 mg/4 h) or by IV infusion (1–2 mg per hour via a central line) to reduce cerebral artery spasm and is thought to reduce mortality. All patients should be discussed with a neurosurgeon.

Resources

NICE *Subarachnoid haemorrhage due to ruptured aneurysms*, draft scope for consultation (2018): www. nice.org.uk/guidance/GID-NG10097/documents/ draft-scope

Case 7: Alcoholic liver disease

👤 Presenting complaint

▸ NH is a 52-year-old gentleman who is known to have alcoholic liver disease. He presented with multiple falls and a general deterioration in his health.

History of presenting complaint

▸ NH has had multiple admissions over the last 4–5 months.

▸ Six months ago, NH went to the pub and says that he drank 1.5 pints of Guinness. He remembers feeling extremely light-headed and he collapsed in the bar. He did not lose consciousness and denies any seizures.

▸ He was then admitted to hospital and found to have postural hypotension.

▸ Since then, NH feels that he has deteriorated, and he has had multiple falls at home. His mobility is very poor and he complains of severe weakness to the point that he can't rise from a chair unassisted.

▸ He says he is passing stools with streaks of blood but denies melaena. He also has a two-week history of diarrhoea.

▸ He appears jaundiced and drowsy. He has lost 3 stone (19 kg) in the past 4–5 months. He attributes this weight loss to poor appetite.

Past medical history

▸ Alcohol dependence, alcoholic liver disease (ALD)

▸ Type 2 diabetes mellitus

▸ Anxiety/depression.

Drug history

Drug	Class	Dose	Frequency	Indication
Metformin	Biguanide	500 mg	×3 (breakfast, lunch, dinner)	Type 2 diabetes
Sertraline	SSRI	100 mg	×1	Depression
Aspirin	COX inhibitor	75 mg	×1	Cardioprotection
Atenolol	Beta-blocker	50 mg	×1	Hypertension
Vitamin B and thiamine	Vitamins	200 mg	×1	Prevent deficiency

(continued overleaf)

Drug	Class	Dose	Frequency	Indication
Simvastatin	HMG-CoA reductase inhibitor	40 mg	×1	Hyperlipidaemia
Furosemide	Loop diuretic	80 mg	×1	Ascites
Lactulose	Osmotic laxative	15 mL	×3	Prevention of hepatic encephalopathy (discourages proliferation of ammonia-producing organisms)
Omeprazole	PPI	20 mg	×1	Gastroprotection

SSRI, selective serotonin reuptake inhibitor; PPI, proton pump inhibitor.

Allergies

▸ NKDA.

Family history

▸ Mother died aged 51 from an MI

▸ Father is in a nursing home (aged 84 years)

▸ NH had a brother who hanged himself. The brother had a history of drug abuse.

Social history

▸ NH's wife has recently been diagnosed with terminal lung cancer and has been given a prognosis of 12 months.

▸ NH is cared for at home by his wife and is struggling to cope at the moment.

▸ He lost his job as a train driver 4 months ago. He had previously been absent from work due to 'depression and falls'. However, NH also acknowledged that he has been drinking excessively for a number of years. His father-in-law, whom NH was very close to, died 3 years ago, and this is when NH believes his drinking escalated.

▸ He has been a heavy drinker for about 10 years and now drinks a bottle of whisky a day.

▸ He is a non-smoker.

Systemic enquiry

▸ **Neurological:** Frequent falls. No LOC, seizures or dizziness. Occasional headaches.

▸ **Cardiovascular:** Ankle oedema and postural hypotension. No chest pain or breathlessness.

▸ **Respiratory:** Nil.

▸ **Genitourinary:** Nil.

▸ **Gastrointestinal:** Generalised abdominal pain. Poor swallowing. Frequent diarrhoea with streaks of blood.

▸ **Musculoskeletal:** Very weak and extremely poor mobility.

Physical examination

General

▸ NH appears drowsy and has a flat appearance. He is seated and is clearly jaundiced.

▸ NH was difficult to examine owing to his poor mobility. He was unable to rise from the chair, so examination was conducted there.

Vital signs

▸ BP 115/59 mmHg

▸ HR 60 bpm – regular

▸ RR 18 breaths/minute.

Gastrointestinal/abdominal

▸ No hepatic flap

▸ Gross ascites; the abdomen is soft with mild tenderness, the liver edge is palpable

▸ Bowel sounds present.

☰ Summary of patient's problems

▸ Alcohol dependence

▸ Alcoholic liver disease (ALD)

▸ Poor mobility

▸ Poor nutritional status.

❷ Questions

▸ Based on the patient's symptoms, what are the main differential diagnoses?

▸ What initial investigations would help confirm the diagnosis?

▸ What is your immediate management plan?

Differential diagnosis

Jaundice and deranged LFTs:

▶ Hepatitis: alcohol/drug-induced; viral (hepatitis A, B, C)

▶ Autoimmune: primary biliary cirrhosis, primary sclerosing cholangitis

▶ Non-alcoholic fatty liver disease (NAFLD)

▶ Haemochromatosis

▶ Obstructive jaundice – secondary to gallstones, pancreatic or biliary malignancy, metastatic disease (think of this in painless jaundice).

Management plan

▶ Assess ABCDE

▶ IV access and bloods

▶ Liver screen:

> liver autoantibodies (AMA/ASMA/ANA/LKM)

> immunoglobulins

> ferritin (+/– *HFE* genotype)

> viral hepatitis serology (A, B, C, E)

> caeruloplasmin, α-1-antitrypsin, coeliac serology, AFP

▶ Abdominal ultrasound – if ascites, consider paracentesis.

Results of investigations

Blood results

Substance	Reference range	Value
Total bilirubin	<20 μmol/L	51 μmol/L
Alk phos	30–130 U/L	433 U/L
AST	10–40 U/L	199 U/L
ALT	10–50 U/L	72 U/L
Albumin	39–51 g/L	36 g/L
Urea	2.5–7.5 mmol/L	1.3 mmol/L
Creatinine	50–125 μmol/L	65 μmol/L
Na$^+$	135–145 mmol/L	144 mmol/L
K$^+$	3.5–5.0 mmol/L	3.1 mmol/L

❓ Questions

▸ What do the blood tests show?

Abdominal ultrasound

Ascites and cirrhotic changes.

Diagnosis

▸ Alcoholic liver disease

This patient's blood results indicate a hepatic picture. Alcohol is the most likely cause in the context of alcohol dependency. Urea and albumin are often also reduced in chronic alcoholics. MCV is usually raised.

Revised management plan

▸ Continue diuretics (furosemide 80 mg)

▸ Spironolactone

▸ Involve dietitians (limit dietary protein as prophylaxis against encephalopathy and reduce sodium intake); monitor weight

▸ Lactulose (prevents bowel ammonia build-up which can lead to hepatic encephalopathy)

▸ Continue with thiamine and vitamin B complex

▸ Advise on alcohol abstinence; discuss options such as Alcoholics Anonymous (AA) and other local support

▸ Physiotherapy.

Background information: alcoholic liver disease

Alcohol is the most common cause of chronic liver disease in the Western world. Alcoholic liver disease is more common in men and usually occurs in the fourth or fifth decade of life. However, increased consumption of alcohol means that now some men are presenting in their 20s and many more women are also seen with the disease.

Alcohol is a hepatotoxin, yet only 10–20% of people who drink excessively will develop cirrhosis, which means that genetic predisposition and immunological mechanisms must also be involved.

There are three major pathological lesions and clinical illnesses associated with excessive alcohol intake.

Alcoholic fatty liver

The metabolism of alcohol produces fat, and with large amounts of alcohol intake, hepatocytes become swollen with fat (steatosis). Alcoholic fatty liver is the most common biopsy finding in people who are dependent on alcohol. It is not associated with liver cell damage, and the liver will return to normal after about 6 weeks with abstinence. There are usually no symptoms but there may be hepatomegaly on examination. Laboratory tests are often normal, yet an elevated MCV is often an early indicator of heavy drinking. Gamma-GT is usually elevated. If the individual continues to consume alcohol, they may develop fibrosis and ultimately cirrhosis.

Alcoholic hepatitis

In addition to fatty change seen in alcoholic fatty liver there is infiltration of polymorphonuclear leukocytes with the accumulation of dense cytoplasmic inclusion bodies which are known as Mallory bodies. Severely damaged hepatocytes become necrotic. Sinusoids and terminal hepatic venules are narrowed. Cirrhosis may also be present.

Individuals may be asymptomatic. However, most are very unwell and undernourished and present with fatigue, fever, jaundice, right upper quadrant pain, and tender hepatomegaly. Investigations reveal a leukocytosis with elevated bilirubin and transferases. However, the AST and ALT levels are usually less than 500 U/L. If they are higher than this, then another cause for the hepatitis should be sought (think paracetamol toxicity or shocked liver).

Alcoholic cirrhosis

Cirrhosis implies irreversible liver damage and is the final and most severe manifestation of chronic alcohol abuse. The liver architecture is diffusely abnormal and this interferes with normal blood flow and function. There is destruction and fibrosis, and nodules resulting from attempted regeneration. Two pathological types of cirrhosis have been described.

▶ Micronodular cirrhosis: regenerating nodules are generally less than 3 mm. This type is most often seen in chronic alcohol abuse or biliary tract disease.

▶ Macronodular cirrhosis: the nodules are of varying size and normal acini may be present.

Patients often present with one of the complications of cirrhosis. These include:

▶ right hypochondrial pain due to liver distension

▶ abdominal distension due to fluid retention

▶ ankle swelling due to fluid retention

▶ haematemesis and melaena from GI haemorrhage

▶ pruritus due to cholestasis – this is often an early symptom of primary biliary cirrhosis

- breast swelling (gynaecomastia), loss of libido and amenorrhoea due to endocrine dysfunction

- confusion and drowsiness due to neuropsychiatric complication (portosystemic encephalopathy)

- ascites – the presence of fluid in the peritoneal cavity, a common complication of cirrhosis of the liver.

Aetiology of ascites

The peripheral vasodilation in cirrhosis leads to a reduction in effective blood volume and activation of the sympathetic nervous system and the renin–angiotensin–aldosterone system, thus promoting salt and water retention.

Oedema is favoured by hypoalbuminaemia and is localised mainly to the peritoneal cavity due to portal hypertension caused by increased hydrostatic pressure that results from sinusoidal damage.

Other causes of ascites include:

Transudate:

- constrictive pericarditis

- cardiac failure

- hypoalbuminaemia, e.g. nephrotic syndrome (triad of proteinuria, hypoalbuminaemia and oedema)

- Meigs' syndrome (ovarian tumour, ascites and hydrothorax).

Exudates:

- malignancy

- infection, e.g. pyogenic, TB, pancreatitis

- Budd–Chiari syndrome (occlusion of the hepatic vein)

- myxoedema

- lymphatic obstruction (chylous ascites).

Management of ascites

- Dietary salt and water restriction (salt intake = 5.2 g/day)

- Diuretics – spironolactone 400 mg per day is preferred for its aldosterone-antagonising properties. Furosemide 20–40 mg is added if the response is poor. The success of diuretic therapy is assessed by measuring daily weights. Aim for therapy to produce loss of 0.5 kg/day.

- Paracentesis – used in patients with tense ascites or who are resistant to medical therapy. The major danger of this approach is hypovolaemia, because the ascites reaccumulates at the expense of normal circulating volume.

Resources

EASL Clinical Practice Guidelines: *Management of alcohol-related liver disease*: https://easl.eu/publication/management-of-alcohol-related-liver-disease/

Case 8: Thirst and fatigue

Presenting complaint

▶ JC is a 78-year-old gentleman who presented with extreme thirst and fatigue.

History of presenting complaint

▶ JC remembers first becoming symptomatic 8 years ago whilst on holiday aboard a cruise ship.

▶ He had an 'unquenchable thirst' and drank excessive amounts of water.

▶ Excessive urination (polyuria).

▶ No weight change.

Past medical history

▶ Cataract

▶ Incontinent of faeces

▶ Haemorrhoids

▶ Transient cerebral ischaemia

▶ Pure hypercholesterolaemia

▶ Chronic kidney disease stage 3

▶ Diverticulosis

▶ Type 2 diabetes mellitus

▶ Essential hypertension

▶ Neurotic depression reactive type

Drug history

Drug	Class	Dose	Frequency	Indication
Levetiracetam	Antiepileptic	250 mg	bd	Epilepsy
Simvastatin	HMG-CoA reductase inhibitor	40 mg	nocte	Hypercholesterolaemia
Metformin	Biguanide	500 mg	2 tabs at bedtime	Type 2 diabetes
Aspirin	COX inhibitor	75 mg	1 tab in morning	Cardioprotection
Paroxetine	SSRI	20 mg	1 tab in morning	Depression

Allergies

▶ NKDA.

Family history

▸ No significant family history

▸ Mother had history of dementia; died aged 80 from 'old age'

▸ Father died in his 50s from complications of a gangrenous leg.

Social history

▸ Formerly married for 7 years but has been divorced for 50 years

▸ No children

▸ JC has been in a monogamous relationship for the last 20 years; the relationship was initially sexual, but JC encounters erection difficulties and the couple have not had a sexual relationship for a number of years

▸ JC worked as a storeman for Scottish Power for 29 years, and is now retired

▸ JC gets very little exercise and spends most of his time at home in front of the television, due to a combination of his depression and his poor mobility

▸ He has smoked 30 cigarettes a day for 60 years (90 pack-year history)

▸ No alcohol

▸ JC says that he is very careful with money and this is reflected in his diet. He eats almost no fruit or vegetables and buys reduced price food.

Systemic enquiry

▸ **Neurological:** Frequent falls, no fits or seizures, no paraesthesia, poor balance.

▸ **Cardiovascular:** Nil.

▸ **Respiratory:** Chronic, persistent, productive cough (yellow sputum). Occasional exertional dyspnoea.

▸ **Genitourinary:** Nocturia (2–3 times per night). Past history of haematuria. No dysuria, urgency or discharge.

▸ **Gastrointestinal:** History of recurrent diarrhoea. No blood or mucus.

▸ **Musculoskeletal:** Poor mobility. He is unable to walk more than 100 metres due to 'tiredness'. No pain or stiffness in any joint.

Physical examination

General

▸ Alert but slightly unkempt, elderly gentleman with an almost expressionless face.

▸ Slow, quiet and monotonous speech.

- No pallor, jaundice, cyanosis or clubbing.
- Tar-stained fingers and palmar erythema.

Vital signs

- Temp 37.6°C
- HR 60 bpm – regular but frequent ectopic beat
- BP 150/92 mmHg
- RR 16 breaths/minute
- BMI 28.7

Neurological

- Patient is orientated to person, time and place
- Motor: good bulk and tone; strength is 5/5 throughout
- Cerebellar: finger–nose, heel–shin and rapid alternating movement responses are intact
- Normal gait.

Cardiovascular

- No visible JVP
- Good S1, S2; no added sounds or murmurs
- Unable to palpate apex beat
- Peripheral pulses present
- No oedema.

Respiratory

- Thorax symmetrical with good expansion
- Slightly dyspnoeic
- Lungs resonant; vesicular breath sounds
- Wheeze.

Gastrointestinal/abdominal

- Soft and non-tender
- Active bowel sounds.

Musculoskeletal

- Full range of movement in all joints; no swelling or deformities
- Walks with an aid.

☰ Summary of patient's problems

- Poorly controlled type 2 diabetes mellitus
- Ongoing depression and social withdrawal
- Chronic kidney disease
- Fatigue and excessive tiredness
- Poor compliance
- Poor diet
- Poor mobility
- Smoker.

Differential diagnosis

Fatigue and polydipsia:

Polydipsia

▸ **Diabetes mellitus**

▸ Hypokalaemia

▸ Hypercalcaemia (polyuria results from the effect of hypercalcaemia on renal tubules, reducing their concentrating ability – a form of mild nephrogenic diabetes insipidus)

▸ Diabetes insipidus

▸ Chronic renal failure

▸ Excessive fluid intake (psychogenic polydipsia).

Fatigue

▸ Anaemia

▸ Infections (Epstein–Barr virus, cytomegalovirus, hepatitis)

▸ Diabetes mellitus

▸ Hypo- or hyperthyroidism

▸ Perimenopausal

▸ Asthma

▸ Sleep apnoea

▸ Depression.

Results of investigations

Blood results

Description	Reference range	Value
FBC		normal
Urea	2.5–7.0 mmol/L	7.6 mmol/L
Creatinine	60–120 µmol/L	65 µmol/L
Glucose	3.0–6.0 mmol/L	23.9 mmol/L **high**
Cholesterol	<5 mmol/L	4.9 mmol/L
TFTs: TSH	0.3–3.5	1.76

> **Diagnosis**
>
> ▶ Type 2 diabetes mellitus
>
> JC presented with fatigue, polydipsia and hyperglycaemia confirming the diagnosis.

Management plan

▶ Lifestyle advice, with focus on diet and exercise

▶ JC has an extremely poor diet which undoubtedly contributes to his poor diabetic control, so he may benefit from a dietitian referral

▶ Achievement of good glycaemic control

▶ Modification of risk factors for vascular disease, i.e. hypertension, hypercholesterolaemia, smoking

▶ JC has consistently high HbA1c readings, suggesting poor compliance, so further education and input from specialised diabetic nurses may improve his situation.

Background information: diabetes mellitus

Diabetes mellitus is characterised by hyperglycaemia. It is the result of insulin deficiency, insulin resistance or both. Globally, an estimated 422 million adults were living with diabetes in 2014, compared to 108 million in 1980 (WHO – Global report on diabetes). It therefore represents a major public health problem.

The chronic hyperglycaemia that occurs in diabetes mellitus is associated with damage to various organ systems and may lead to macrovascular disease, and thence to increased prevalence of coronary artery disease, peripheral vascular disease and stroke. Microvascular complications include diabetic retinopathy, nephropathy and neuropathy.

Clinical classification

Diabetes mellitus may be classified into two types.

▶ type 1 diabetes – absolute insulin deficiency, where insulin therapy is necessary for survival

▶ type 2 diabetes – insulin resistance or relative insulin deficiency, where control of blood glucose levels may be achieved by lifestyle or oral medications; however, insulin may be required in those with uncontrolled type 2 diabetes (glycated haemoglobin [HbA1c] >7.5–8.0% on maximum oral therapy).

Comparison of type 1 and type 2 diabetes

	Type 1 diabetes mellitus	Type 2 diabetes mellitus
Epidemiology	Younger patients	Older patients
Genetics	HLA-DR3 and -DR4 linked	No HLA association

	Type 1 diabetes mellitus	Type 2 diabetes mellitus
Aetiology	Autoimmune beta-cell destruction	Peripheral insulin resistance beta cell dysfunction
Presentation	Polydipsia, polyuria, weight loss, ketoacidosis	Often asymptomatic; presents with macro- and microvascular complications

HLA, human leukocyte antigen.

Background information: type 1 diabetes mellitus (insulin dependent)

Epidemiology

▶ Younger (usually <30 years old)

▶ Usually lean.

Heredity

▶ HLA-DR3 or -DR4 in >90%

▶ 30–50% concordance in identical twins.

Pathogenesis

▶ Autoimmune disease: insulin deficiency due to selective destruction of insulin-secreting pancreatic beta cells

▶ Associated with other autoimmune diseases.

Clinical

▶ Insulin deficiency

▶ May develop ketoacidosis

▶ Weight loss

▶ Always need insulin.

Background information: type 2 diabetes mellitus

Epidemiology

This is a common disease in affluent countries. There are four major determinants:

▶ increasing age

▶ obesity

▶ ethnicity

▶ family history.

The prevalence in the UK is approximately 2%, yet it is 2–3 times more prevalent in people of South Asian, African and Caribbean ancestry. Most individuals are over the age of 40 but more teenagers are increasingly being seen with type 2 diabetes mellitus secondary to increasing obesity levels.

The insulin-resistant state seen in type 2 diabetes is commonly seen in conjunction with other conditions which increase cardiovascular risk. These include: hypertension, obesity, hypercholesterolaemia, decreased HDL (high-density lipoprotein) cholesterol and the skin condition acanthosis nigricans (thickened, hyperpigmented skin at flexures, usually due to excess insulin in obese individuals or in malignancy). This is called **insulin resistance syndrome**, **syndrome X** or **metabolic syndrome**. It is related to exercise, lifestyle and body weight.

Aetiology

There is a strong genetic tendency to type 2 diabetes, which is much greater than in type 1. There is a 50% concordance in identical twins. However, many of the genes remain unknown.

Obesity is the major environmental factor predisposing to type 2 diabetes, and is thought to have a role in insulin resistance, possibly because of down-regulation of insulin receptors due to hyperinsulinaemia.

Clinical presentation

Type 2 diabetes may go undiagnosed for many years. An elevated blood glucose level may therefore be present for many years before diagnosis, resulting in secondary complications. Patients may be identified by the finding of an elevated plasma glucose level. Despite this, 50% of patients are identified when they present with some of the classical symptoms (polyuria, polydipsia, blurred vision) or recurrent infections (staphylococcal skin infections, *Candida*-related balanitis or pruritus vulvae), or with fatigue and malaise.

Diagnosis

WHO diagnostic criteria (WHO, 2006)	
Normoglycaemia	Fasting plasma glucose <6.1 mmol/L
	OR 2 hour post-75 g load plasma glucose <7.8 mmol/L
Diabetes	Random plasma glucose >11.1 mmol/L
	OR Fasting plasma glucose >7.0 mmol/L
	OR 2 hour post-75 g load plasma glucose >11.1 mmol/L
Impaired glucose tolerance	2 hour post-75 g load plasma glucose 7.8–11.1 mmol/L
Gestational diabetes	Random plasma glucose >11.1 mmol/L (200 mg/dL)
	OR Fasting plasma glucose > 6.0 mmol/L
	OR 2 hour post-75 g load plasma glucose >7.8 mmol/L*

Management

Enabling patients to manage their own condition by education and with motivation from a multidisciplinary team is central to successful treatment.

Diet

Diet is the mainstay of treatment and newly diagnosed patients should have a 3-month trial of diet therapy alone unless:

▶ they are severely symptomatic

▶ their blood glucose level is consistently greater than 20 mmol/L.

Lifestyle modification

In order to prevent secondary complications from diabetes, lifestyle modifications are imperative. Patients should be educated on the beneficial effects of exercise on their diabetes and should also be encouraged to stop smoking. JC's history of depression and poor mobility inhibit his ability to exercise and further complicate the case. He has also expressed an unwillingness to stop smoking.

Medication

Oral hypoglycaemics include:

▶ Biguanides increase insulin sensitivity and maintain weight loss
  > side-effects nausea and diarrhoea often transient; no hypoglycaemia
  > avoid if creatinine >150 μmol/L because of risk of lactic acidosis
  > e.g. metformin.

▶ Sulphonylureas increase insulin secretion
  > side-effects hypoglycaemia, weight gain
  > e.g. tolbutamide, gliclazide, glibenclamide.

▶ Thiazolidinediones increase insulin sensitivity
  > side-effects hypoglycaemia, fluid retention, hepatotoxicity
  > e.g. pioglitazone, rosiglitazone.

If metformin is contraindicated or not tolerated, consider initial drug treatment with a dipeptidyl peptidase-4 (DPP-4) inhibitor or pioglitazone or a sulphonylurea.

Do not give pioglitazone to adults with type 2 diabetes if they have any of the following:

▶ heart failure or history of heart failure

▶ hepatic impairment

▶ diabetic ketoacidosis

▶ current, or a history of, bladder cancer

▶ uninvestigated macroscopic haematuria.

Treatment with sodium–glucose cotransporter 2 (SGLT-2) inhibitors may be appropriate if metformin is not an option.

In type 2 diabetes, several factors have been shown to be associated with a poor level of compliance, such as age, diabetes duration, low socioeconomic level, presence of complications, polypharmacy, and multiple daily dosing of antidiabetic oral agents. Further education and input from specialised diabetic nurses may help.

Resources

NICE *Type 2 diabetes in adults: management: NG28* (2017): www.nice.org.uk/guidance/ng28/resources

WHO *Definition and diagnosis of diabetes mellitus and intermediate hyperglycaemia: Report of a WHO/IDF consultation* (2006): www.who.int/diabetes/publications/diagnosis_diabetes2006/en/

Case 9: Deteriorating vision

Presenting complaint

▸ JP is a 74-year-old gentleman who presented with deteriorating vision in his right eye.

History of presenting complaint

▸ Five months ago, JP noticed that his vision was deteriorating in his right eye.

▸ He describes it as a blurring of his vision that gradually occurred over a period of months.

▸ JP felt that he needed glasses and went to his optician.

▸ The optician noticed retinal changes and referred JP to his GP.

▸ At this stage, JP was found to have significant retinal changes associated with hypertension.

▸ His BP was 200/80 mmHg.

▸ He has occasional headaches.

▸ No ocular pain.

Past medical history

▸ Transient ischaemic attack

▸ Pulmonary tuberculosis (TB)

▸ Arthroscopy

▸ Stroke

▸ Endarterectomy

▸ Bilateral vasectomy for contraception

Drug history

Drug	Class	Dose	Frequency	Indication
Atenolol	Beta-blocker	25 mg	1 tab in the morning	Hypertension
Amlodipine	Calcium channel blocker	5 mg	1 tab in the morning	Hypertension
Ramipril	ACE inhibitor	2.5 mg	2 caps daily	Hypertension
Daktacort	Hydrocortisone	Apply sparingly	tds	Candida intertrigo
Simvastatin	Statin	20 mg	1 tab at night	Hyperlipidaemia

Allergies

▸ NKDA.

Family history

▶ Mother died aged 62 from bowel cancer

▶ Father died aged 73 from 'natural causes'

▶ Significant family history of cardiovascular disease: JP has 6 sisters, all of whom have hypertension

▶ One of his sisters has a history of myocardial infarction and another has a pacemaker.

Social history

▶ JP has been married for 51 years. He says his wife is in 'great health'.

▶ They have two daughters (aged 49 and 47). Both are healthy.

▶ He has two grandchildren (aged 23 and 21 years).

▶ JP and his wife have lived in the same house for 42 years. It is a semi-detached house with two storeys.

▶ JP now finds the stairs a problem because of pain in his right knee which is a consequence of recurrent cycling accidents.

▶ He was a member of a cycling club for many years, giving up a few years ago due to injury.

▶ Worked with Rolls Royce as an engineer for 33 years. His wife previously worked part-time as a secretary. Both are now retired.

▶ JP says that he is financially comfortable.

▶ He plays golf three times a week.

▶ JP smokes 15 cigarettes a day. He has no intention of stopping as he feels that it is not adversely affecting his health.

▶ He used to drink a moderate amount of alcohol but has not drunk in over 30 years.

▶ He feels that he has a healthy, balanced diet.

Systemic enquiry

▶ **Neurological:** Deteriorating vision in his right eye.

▶ **Cardiovascular:** No chest pain, palpitations or breathlessness.

▶ **Respiratory:** Nil.

▶ **Genitourinary:** Nil.

▶ **Gastrointestinal:** Nil.

▶ **Musculoskeletal:** Pain in right knee.

Physical examination

General

▸ Alert, sitting comfortably upright and in no obvious pain or discomfort

▸ No pallor, jaundice, cyanosis or clubbing.

Vital signs

▸ BP 142/92 mmHg   ▸ RR 16 breaths/minute

▸ HR 52 bpm – normal rate, rhythm, volume and character.

Cardiovascular

▸ No visible JVP

▸ Unable to palpate apex beat

▸ S1, S2; regular rate; loud ejection systolic murmur

▸ Peripheral pulses present

▸ No oedema.

Genitourinary

▸ Unable to palpate the kidneys.

Fundoscopy

▸ Extensive dot and blot haemorrhages and exudates.

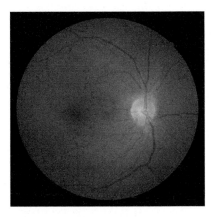

☰ Summary of patient's problems

▸ Hypertension

▸ Smoker

▸ Hypertensive retinopathy.

❷ Questions

▸ What are the main differential diagnoses of gradual visual loss?

▸ What initial investigations would help confirm the diagnosis?

▸ What is your immediate management plan?

▸ According to the Keith–Wagener classification, what grade of retinopathy does JP have?

Differential diagnosis

Gradual vision loss:

▸ Diabetic retinopathy

▸ Hypertensive retinopathy

▸ Cataract (lens opacity) – most common cause of blindness in the world today

▸ Age-related macular degeneration – may occur gradually and is typified by loss of the central field

▸ Choroiditis

▸ Choroid melanoma – most common malignant tumour of the eye, causes retinal detachment

▸ Optic atrophy – optic disc is pale. May be secondary to increased intraocular pressure (in glaucoma) or retinal damage (as in choroiditis, retinitis pigmentosa, cerebromacular degeneration), or due to ischaemia (as in retinal artery occlusion).

Investigations

▸ Urinalysis – look for diabetes (glucose), protein and blood

▸ ECG – look for myocardial ischaemia, left ventricular hypertrophy

▸ U+Es – for evaluation of renal impairment, hyperaldosteronism (Conn's syndrome – increased BP with decreased potassium)

▸ Fasting blood for lipids (total and HDL cholesterol) and glucose

▸ TFTs.

Results of investigations

▸ Urinalysis:

> urine creatinine 10.32 mmol/L

> urine albumin 223.0 mg/L

> albumin/creatinine 21.6 mg/mmol (reference 0–2.5 mg/mmol)

> proteinuria

▸ Urea 11 mmol/L (2.5–7.0 mmol/L)

▸ Creatinine 163 μmol/L (60–120 μmol/L)

▸ Estimated glomerular filtration rate (eGFR) 37 mL/min (90–140 mL/min) – U+Es illustrate chronic kidney disease

▸ ECG showed left ventricular hypertrophy

▸ Cholesterol 4.1 mmol/L

▸ Cholesterol/HDL ratio 4.6 mmol/L

▸ TSH 2.1 mU/L (0.15–4.0 mU/L).

Diagnosis

▶ Retinopathy due to essential hypertension

This patient presented with deteriorating vision in his right eye. He was hypertensive and fundoscopy confirmed grade 3 retinopathy.

Management plan

▶ Weight reduction – BMI should be <25 kg/m^2

▶ Low-fat and low-saturated-fat diet

▶ Low-sodium diet – <6 g NaCl per day

▶ Limited alcohol consumption

▶ Dynamic exercise – at least 30 minutes' brisk walk per day

▶ Increased fruit and vegetable consumption

▶ Reduce cardiovascular risk by stopping smoking and increasing oily fish consumption

▶ Pharmacological: initiation of antihypertensive therapy.

Background information: hypertension

Hypertension is a major cause of premature vascular disease leading to cerebrovascular events such as stroke and myocardial infarctions. Hypertension is typically asymptomatic until it causes organ damage, thus screening is vital. All adults should have their BP measured routinely at least every 5 years until the age of 80 years.

Classification of blood pressure levels (British Hypertension Society)

Category	Systolic BP (mmHg)	Diastolic (mmHg)
Optimal	<120	<80
Normal	<130	<85
High normal	130–139	85–89
Hypertension:		
Grade 1 (mild)	140–159	90–99
Grade 2 (moderate)	160–179	100–109
Grade 3 (severe)	>180	>110
Isolated systolic hypertension		
Grade 1	140–159	<90
Grade 2	>160	<90

Causes

In approximately 95% of cases, the cause of hypertension is unknown – **essential hypertension**. Essential hypertension has a multifactorial aetiology.

Genetic factors

Hypertension has a tendency to run in families; however, the genes responsible have still to be identified. JP believes this is the reason for his hypertension as he does have a very strong family history.

Environmental factors

▶ Obesity

▶ Excessive alcohol intake

▶ High sodium intake

▶ Stress.

Hypertension attributed to a definable cause is termed **secondary hypertension**. Conditions that cause secondary hypertension are far less common than essential hypertension, but they are important as they are amenable to permanent cure.

Causes of secondary hypertension

▶ Renal disease (most common secondary cause) – 75% are from intrinsic renal disease: glomerulonephritis, polyarteritis nodosa (PAN), systemic sclerosis, chronic pyelonephritis or polycystic kidneys. The remaining 25% are due to renovascular disease, most commonly atheromatous or rarely fibromuscular dysplasia.

▶ Endocrine disease: Cushing's, Conn's (aldosterone-producing tumour), phaeochromocytoma, acromegaly, hyperparathyroidism.

▶ Other: Pregnancy, steroids, the contraceptive pill.

Malignant hypertension refers to severe hypertension (systolic >200, diastolic >130 mmHg). Unless treated it may lead to death from progressive renal failure, heart failure, aortic dissection or stroke. JP presented initially with a BP reading of 200/80 mmHg. He also had signs of progressive renal failure and proteinuria. Typically, in the retina there may be flame-shaped haemorrhages, cotton-wool spots, hard exudates and papilloedema. JP did indeed have many of these classical signs, with his only symptom being progressive visual disturbance.

Hypertensive retinopathy is a condition characterised by a spectrum of retinal vascular signs in people with elevated BP.

The retinal circulation undergoes a series of pathophysiological changes in response to elevated BP. In the initial vasoconstrictive stage, there is vasospasm and an increase in retinal arteriolar tone owing to local autoregulatory mechanisms. This stage is seen clinically as a generalised narrowing of the retinal arterioles. Persistently elevated BP leads to intimal thickening, hyperplasia of the media wall, and then hyaline degeneration in the subsequent, sclerotic, stage. This stage corresponds to more severe generalised and focal areas of arteriolar narrowing, changes in the arteriolar and venular junctions (i.e., arteriovenous nicking or nipping), and alterations in the arteriolar light reflex (increased reflection of light through the ophthalmoscope, termed 'copper wiring' or 'silver wiring').

This is followed by an exudative stage, in which there is disruption of the blood–retina barrier, necrosis of the smooth muscles and endothelial cells, exudation of blood and lipids, and retinal ischaemia. These changes are manifested in the retina as microaneurysms, haemorrhages, hard exudates and cotton-wool spots. Swelling of the optic disc may occur at this time and usually indicates severely elevated BP (i.e. malignant hypertension).

The abnormalities are graded according to the Keith–Wagener classification.

▶ Grade 1 – Tortuous arteries with thick shiny walls ('silver wiring' or 'copper wiring').

▶ Grade 2 – AV nipping (narrowing where arteries cross veins).

▶ Grade 3 – Flame-shaped haemorrhages and cotton-wool spots.

▶ Grade 4 – Papilloedema.

Management

All patients with malignant hypertension or a sustained pressure >160/100 mmHg should be treated. For those with BP >140/90 mmHg,

the decision to treat depends on the risk of coronary events, presence of diabetes or end-organ damage.

The treatment goal is to achieve a BP of <140/85 mmHg, but in diabetes, aim for <130/80 mmHg and <125/75 mmHg if proteinuria is present.

The management of hypertension involves lifestyle modifications, as outlined above, and pharmacological measures.

It is important to explain to the patient that long-term treatment is needed. An explanation of the benefits of treatment may help to improve compliance.

The NICE guidelines (CG127, 2016) state that:

▶ If patient >55 years old, and in black patients of any age, first choice is a calcium channel blocker or thiazide.

▶ If <55 years, first choice is an ACE inhibitor.

▶ If initial treatment was with a calcium channel blocker or thiazide, and a second drug is needed, add an ACE inhibitor. If initial treatment was with an ACE inhibitor, add a calcium channel blocker or a thiazide.

▶ If treatment with three drugs is needed, try ACE inhibitor, calcium channel blocker and thiazide.

▶ If BP is still uncontrolled, add a fourth drug and seek help.

Resources

European Society of Cardiology/ESH *Clinical Practice Guidelines: Arterial hypertension* (2018): www.escardio.org/Guidelines/Clinical-Practice-Guidelines/Arterial-Hypertension-Management-of

NICE *Hypertension in adults: diagnosis and management: Clinical guideline 127* (2016): www.nice.org.uk/guidance/cg127

Chapter 2:

Surgery

Case 10: Abdominal pain

Presenting complaint

▶ SG is a 40-year-old gentleman who presented with acute abdominal pain.

History of presenting complaint

▶ SG presented with a 36-hour history of abdominal pain. Initially the pain was localised to the epigastric region, but went on to radiate to the umbilicus and then to the right iliac fossa. The pain was severe and was aggravated by movement.

▶ He describes the pain as the worst he has ever experienced. It was not associated with nausea or vomiting. He had no appetite and was unable to eat or drink anything.

▶ His bowels had opened on the day of admission and he did not notice any rectal PR bleeding or melaena.

▶ He presented to his GP, who made a referral to the surgeon.

▶ A few hours after admission, SG began to show signs of peritonism with severe generalised abdominal pain, fever and tachycardia.

Past medical history

▶ Nil.

Drug history

▶ Nil.

Allergies

▶ NKDA.

Family history

▶ No significant family history.

▶ His father is 71 years old and has hypertension.

▶ His mother died at the age of 73 as a result of gastric carcinoma.

Social history

▸ SG has been married to his wife for 20 years. They have a 9-year-old daughter and a 17-year-old son. Unfortunately, last year their oldest son died at the age of 18. He had a history of cerebral palsy and other comorbidities.

▸ The death of his son has understandably placed considerable strain on him and his family.

▸ He works as an army officer for the Ministry of Defence.

▸ He is a non-smoker and drinks about 8 units per week.

Systemic enquiry

▸ **Neurological:** Nil.

▸ **Cardiovascular:** Nil.

▸ **Respiratory:** Nil.

▸ **Genitourinary:** Nil.

▸ **Gastrointestinal:** GORD.

▸ **Musculoskeletal:** Nil.

Physical examination

General

▸ Middle-aged gentleman who is pale, very distressed and obviously in severe pain.

Vital signs

▸ Temp 37.6°C

▸ HR 95 bpm – regular

▸ O_2 sats 100% on air.

▸ BP 170/100 mmHg

▸ RR 14 breaths/minute

Cardiovascular

▸ No visible JVP

▸ Apex beat in fifth intercostal space in the mid-clavicular line

▸ S1, S2; regular rate

▸ Peripheral pulses present

▸ No oedema.

Respiratory

▸ Chest clear

▸ No added sounds or wheeze.

Gastrointestinal/abdominal

▸ Right iliac fossa (RIF) tenderness

▸ Guarding and rebound tenderness

▸ Tender to percussion

▸ Bowel sounds active.

☰ Summary of patient's problems

▸ Acute abdominal pain
▸ Fever and tachycardia
▸ Reduced oral intake
▸ Peritonism.

❷ Questions

▸ Based on the patient's symptoms, what are the main differential diagnoses?
▸ What initial investigations would help confirm the diagnosis?
▸ What is your immediate management plan?

Differential diagnosis

▶ Acute perforated appendicitis

▶ Upper GI perforation

▶ Acute perforated diverticular disease

▶ Acute peritonitis.

Initial management plan

▶ Assess ABCDE

▶ Establish IV access

▶ IV fluids

▶ Request bloods (FBC, U+Es, LFTs, CRP, amylase)

▶ Morphine (5 mg IV)

▶ CXR to look for air under the diaphragm (indicative of ruptured viscus)

▶ Nil by mouth (NBM).

Results of investigations

Blood results

Substance	Reference range	Result
Na^+	135–145 mmol/L	137 mmol/l
K^+	3.5–5.0 mmol/L	3.9 mmol/L
Cl^-	97–107 mmol/L	105 mmol/L
HCO_3^-	23–30 mmol/L	18 mmol/L
Urea	2.5–6.7 mmol/L	3.9 mmol/L
Creatinine	40–130 µmol/L	66 µmol/L
Bilirubin	3–17 µmol/L	51 µmol/L
ALT	3–35 U/L	19 U/L
AST	3–35 U/L	19 U/L
Alk phos	40–150 U/L	43 U/L
Hb	115–165 g/L	137 g/L
WCC	$4–11 \times 10^9$/L	11.8×10^9/L
CRP	<10 mg/L	129 mg/L

CXR

Pneumoperitoneum.

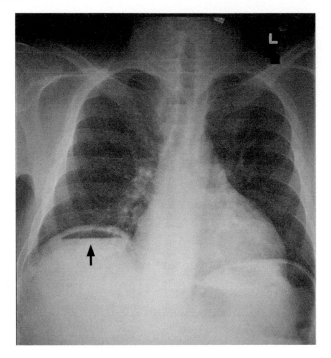

Diagnosis

▶ Acute perforated appendicitis

This 40-year-old gentleman presented with abdominal pain. Initially the pain was localised to the epigastric region but progressed to the RIF. This is typical of appendicitis. The pain was severe and was aggravated by movement. He felt generally unwell and feverish.

Further management plan

An emergency laparoscopy revealed a ruptured appendicitis.

Management involved an appendicectomy and postoperative analgesia and supportive care.

Background information: acute appendicitis

Acute abdominal pain is defined as abdominal pain of less than one week's duration, requiring admission to hospital, which has not been previously investigated or treated. Acute abdominal pain is the most common emergency presentation to hospitals in the UK. It has been estimated that at least 50% of general surgical admissions are emergencies, and of these, 50% present with acute abdominal pain.

Acute abdomen – causes

Surgical	Medical	Gynaecological
Inflammation	**GI**	▸ ectopic pregnancy
▸ inflammatory bowel disease	▸ gastritis	▸ ovarian cyst
▸ acute appendicitis	▸ gastroenteritis	▸ torsion
▸ acute diverticulitis	▸ mesenteric adenitis	▸ rupture
▸ acute pancreatitis	▸ hepatitis	▸ haemorrhage
▸ acute cholecystitis	▸ hepatic abscess	▸ infarction
▸ acute cholangitis	▸ Fitz-Hugh–Curtis syndrome (inflammation of the liver capsule associated with genital tract infection)	▸ infection
▸ Meckel's diverticulitis		▸ PID
Obstruction		▸ fibroid degeneration
▸ intestinal obstruction	▸ primary peritonitis	▸ salpingitis
▸ biliary colic	**Genitourinary**	▸ mittelschmerz
▸ ureteric colic	▸ UTI	▸ endometriosis
▸ acute retention of urine	▸ pyelonephritis	
Perforation	**Cardiovascular**	
▸ perforated peptic ulcer disease	▸ MI	
▸ perforated diverticular disease	**Neurological**	
▸ perforated appendix	▸ tabes dorsalis	
▸ toxic megacolon with perforation	**Haematological**	
▸ perforated bowel	▸ sickle-cell disease	
▸ ruptured AAA	▸ malaria	
	▸ hereditary spherocytosis	
	Endocrine	
	▸ diabetes mellitus	
	▸ thyrotoxicosis	
	▸ Addison's disease	
	Metabolic	
	▸ uraemia	
	▸ hypercalcaemia	
	▸ porphyria	
	Infective	
	▸ herpes zoster	

AAA, abdominal aortic aneurysm; PID, pelvic inflammatory disease.

Acute appendicitis

The appendix is a worm-shaped blind-ending tube that arises from the posteromedial wall of the caecum ~2 cm below the ileocaecal valve. The position of the appendix can be located on the surface of the abdomen at McBurney's point, which is located one-third of the way along a line drawn between the right anterior superior iliac spine and the umbilicus. It has its own mesentery, the mesoappendix, and its blood supply comes from the appendicular artery, a branch of the ileocolic artery.

Epidemiology

Acute appendicitis is the most common cause of urgent abdominal surgery and the most common provisional diagnosis of all surgical admissions in the UK. It is uncommon in patients below the age of 2 and above the age of 65, and is most common in the under-40s, with a peak incidence between 8 and 14.

Aetiology

The aetiology of acute appendicitis remains unclear. A diet lacking in fibre has been implicated, as have infective agents.

Pathogenesis

The cause of acute appendicitis is thought to be obstruction of the appendicular lumen by a mass of inspissated faeces (faecolith), lymphoid hyperplasia, foreign bodies, carcinoid tumours and strictures.

Following obstruction, the wall of the appendix becomes inflamed. Inflammation of the wall of the appendix causes venous congestion, which may compromise arterial flow, leading to ischaemia and infarction.

Differential diagnosis

Children	Adults	Older adults
Non-specific abdominal pain including 'mesenteric adenitis'	Terminal ileal pathology (Crohn's, Meckel's diverticulitis, gastroenteritis)	Ileocaecal pathology (caecal diverticulitis, caecal tumours)
Meckel's diverticulitis	Retroperitoneal pathology (pancreatitis, renal colic)	Colonic pathology (sigmoid diverticulitis)
Ovarian cyst/menstrual symptoms (perimenarchal girls)	Ovarian pathology	Ovarian pathology (cysts, infection, tumours)

Clinical features

Symptoms:

▸ Malaise, anorexia and fever

▸ Diarrhoea is common and may be mistaken for acute gastroenteritis

▸ Abdominal pain starts centrally and localises to the RIF

▸ Abdominal pain caused by coughing and moving.

Signs:

▸ Fever, tachycardia

▸ Abdominal tenderness: peritonism suggests perforation; often maximal over McBurney's point

▸ Palpation in LIF causes pain worse in RIF (Rovsing's sign).

Emergency management

Resuscitation:

▸ Establish IV access

▸ Catheterise and place on a fluid balance chart if hypotensive

▸ Analgesia – morphine (5–10 mg IV)

▸ Request bloods.

Diagnosis:

▸ Diagnosis is usually clinical

▸ Investigations include: abdominal ultrasound, CT, laparoscopy.

Definitive management

Open or laparoscopic appendicectomy.

Resources

ASGBI *Acute abdominal pain* (2014): www.rcseng.ac.uk/-/media/files/rcs/library-and publications/non-journal-publications/emergency-general-surgery--commissioning-guide.pdf

Case 11: Bowel cancer

Presenting complaint

▶ RF is a 71-year-old gentleman who was diagnosed with bowel cancer in March. He was admitted for an elective laparoscopic hemicolectomy.

History of presenting complaint

▶ Bowel screening in Feb was positive for faecal occult blood (FOB). Colonoscopy in March revealed a very tortuous sigmoid colon and a lobulated mass lesion in the ascending colon.

▶ RF says that he had no symptoms. He did not experience any abdominal pain, change in bowel habit, melaena, PR bleeding or weight loss.

▶ However, 2 days before he was admitted for an elective right hemicolectomy, he says that he was in 'agony' due to pain in his right upper quadrant. He says that the pain was severe and rated it as 9/10.

▶ The pain was constant but was getting progressively more severe. It limited his daily activities considerably. He felt that the pain improved if he lay on his right-hand side.

▶ He had not opened his bowels/passed flatus for 3 days. He had not passed urine for 48 hours. On admission, his abdomen was very tender and distended.

Past medical history

▶ AF
▶ Hypertension.
▶ Hypothyroidism

Drug history

Drug	Class	Dose	Frequency	Indication
Warfarin	Vitamin K antagonist	Depends on INR (6 mg)	od	AF
Thyroxine	Thyroid hormone	75 mcg	od	Hypothyroid
Simvastatin	HMG-CoA reductase inhibitor	20 mg	nocte	Hyperlipidaemia
Ramipril	ACE inhibitor	1.25 mg	od	Hypertension
GTN	Nitrate	400 mg	1–2 sprays	Angina prophylaxis
Bisoprolol	Beta-blocker	1.25 mg	od	Heart failure
Nicorandil	Potassium-channel activator	20 mg	bd	Angina prophylaxis

Allergies

▸ Penicillin.

Family history

▸ RF's mother died in her 80s, while his father died aged 64. Both died from MIs.

▸ He has four sisters, all of whom died of 'old age'.

▸ He does not think that there is a family history of cancer.

Social history

▸ RF lives with his wife of 46 years. They have no children.

▸ He previously worked as a pattern-maker, but had to retire early at the age of 59 as a result of osteoarthritis in his right wrist.

▸ He smokes 8 cigarettes/day. He has smoked for 56 years (22 pack-years).

▸ He does not drink alcohol.

Systemic enquiry

▸ **Neurological:** No headaches, weakness or paraesthesia. Occasional postural hypotension.

▸ **Cardiovascular:** Occasional chest pains; no SOB.

▸ **Respiratory:** No cough; no haemoptysis.

▸ **Genitourinary:** Nil.

▸ **Gastrointestinal:** Nil.

▸ **Musculoskeletal:** Osteoarthritis in his right wrist.

Physical examination

General

▸ Elderly gentleman who is pale and obviously in severe pain.

Vital signs

▸ BP 90/60 mmHg   ▸ HR 100 bpm – regularly irregular   ▸ RR 14 breaths/minute.

Gastrointestinal/abdominal

▸ Abdomen is very tender and distended

▸ 'Board-like' generalised rigidity with marked guarding and tenderness.

☰ Summary of patient's problems

▶ Known colon cancer.

▶ Acute deterioration – peritonism.

❓ Questions

▶ Based on the patient's symptoms, what are the main differential diagnoses?

▶ What initial investigations would help confirm the diagnosis?

▶ What is your immediate management plan?

Differential diagnosis

▶ Perforated caecal tumour

▶ Acute perforated appendicitis

▶ Acute perforated diverticular disease

▶ Bowel obstruction.

Results of investigations

Blood results

Substance	Reference range	Result
Na$^+$ (135–145)	135–145 mmol/L	129 mmol/L
K$^+$	3.5–5.0 mmol/L	4.6 mmol/L
Urea	2.5–6.7 mmol/L	24.2 mmol/L
Creatinine	70–150 µmol/L	184 µmol/L
Bilirubin	3–17 µmol/L	21 µmol/L
ALT	3–35 U/L	11 U/L
AST	3–35 U/L	24 U/L
Gamma-GT	11–51 U/L	12 U/L
Alk phos	40–150 U/L	52 U/L
Hb	130–180 g/L	109 g/L
WCC	4–11 × 10^9/L	8.49 × 10^9/L
CRP	<10 mg/L	309 mg/L
INR	2.0–2.5	1.5

❷ Questions

▶ What do the blood tests show?

CXR

There is free air under the right hemidiaphragm consistent with perforation of a hollow viscus (see CXR in case 10).

Diagnosis

▶ Peritonitis secondary to perforated caecal tumour

RF is a 71-year-old gentleman who had been diagnosed with bowel cancer. He exhibited 'board-like' generalised rigidity with marked guarding and tenderness. Bloods revealed an acute kidney injury, mild anaemia and marked inflammatory response. CXR revealed free air under the right hemidiaphragm consistent with perforation of a hollow viscus. An emergency laparotomy was indicative of a perforated caecal tumour.

Management plan

▶ Establish large-calibre IV access and take bloods (including cultures and group and save).

▶ Analgesia and antiemetic

▶ Catheterise and start on a fluid balance chart

▶ Right hemicolectomy and end ileostomy.

Background information: colorectal carcinoma

Colorectal adenocarcinoma is the most common GI malignancy and is second only to lung cancer as a cause of cancer death in westernised countries. Scotland has one of the highest incidences of colorectal cancer in the world (41 per 100 000 in men, and 29 per 100 000 in women). Despite there being an increase in the incidence of colorectal cancer in recent years, the age-standardised mortality from the disease has decreased over the last 20 years, indicating an improvement in prognosis.

In the UK the lifetime risk of colorectal cancer is 5.1%, resulting in 32 000 cases each year. The peak age of incidence is between the ages of 45 and 65, although it is increasing in younger patients.

Aetiology

Diet

A diet high in fibre is associated with lower cancer rates in certain populations, whereas the consumption of a diet high in fat and red meat is associated with increased rates. Furthermore, over 20 studies have consistently found a positive link between obesity and colon cancer.

Smoking, alcohol and exercise

Smoking, alcohol and a lack of exercise are associated with an increased risk of developing colon cancer.

Inflammatory bowel disease

There is an increased risk of colon cancer in those with chronic ulcerative colitis and colonic Crohn's disease.

Genetics

Approximately 35% of all colorectal cancers are thought to have a genetic component. Thus, incidence is increased in those with a strong family history of colonic carcinoma.

The polyposis syndromes also predispose to colorectal cancer. **Familial adenomatous polyposis (FAP)** is one of the most common single-gene disorders predisposing to colorectal cancer. It is inherited as an autosomal dominant trait; the gene responsible is the APC gene, which is located on the long arm of chromosome 5. Polyps usually develop during the teenage years, and symptoms such as bleeding and diarrhoea are usually evident by 21 years. The risk of developing carcinoma is virtually 100% within 15 years if prophylactic colectomy is not undertaken.

The more common autosomal dominant syndrome, **hereditary non-polyposis colorectal cancer (HNPCC)**, accounts for 5% of all cases of colorectal carcinoma. HNPCC is associated with other malignancies such as endometrial, gastric, ovarian, upper urinary tract and small intestine. The minimum criteria for HNPCC diagnosis are:

▶ three or more relatives with histologically proven colorectal cancer, one being a first-degree relative of the other two

▶ two or more generations affected

▶ at least one family member affected before the age of 50.

HNPCC is due to a gene mutation affecting DNA mismatch repair. Mutations are most common in *hMSH2* on chromosome 2p and *hMLH2* on chromosome 2q.

Pathology and staging

The predominant type is adenocarcinoma. Other subtypes include mucinous, signet ring cell, and anaplastic. Colorectal carcinoma may be polypoidal, ulcerating and stenosing. Approximately 75% of tumours are found on the left-hand side of the colon and rectum (rectum, 45%; descending/sigmoid colon, 30%; transverse, 5%; right-sided; 20%). Tumour differentiation may be classified as good, moderate or poor. Tumours can be further assessed using Duke's and TNM staging systems.

Duke's staging for colorectal cancer

Duke's staging		Approx. % 5-year survival
A	Confined to bowel wall only	75–95
B	Spread through bowel wall	55–75
C	Spread to involve lymph nodes	30–60
D	Distant metastases	5–10

Clinical features

Rectal location:

▶ PR bleeding: deep red on the surface of stools.

▶ Change in bowel habit: difficulty with defecation, sensation of incomplete evacuation, and painful defecation (tenesmus).

Descending/sigmoid colon:

▶ PR bleeding: typically dark red, mixed with stool, sometimes clotted.

▶ Change in bowel habit: increased frequency, variable consistency, mucus PR, bloating, flatulence.

Right-sided:

▶ Iron-deficiency anaemia may be the only elective presentation.

Emergency presentations:

Up to 40% of colorectal carcinomas will present as emergencies:

▶ Large-bowel obstruction (colicky pain, bloating, constipation)

▶ Perforation with peritonitis

▶ PR bleeding.

Diagnosis and investigations

▶ PR exam

▶ Barium enema

▶ Colonoscopy.

Preoperative staging of colonic cancer requires thoracoabdominal CT scanning.

Treatment

Preoperative

The bowel is cleared with enemas and oral stimulant laxatives such as Picolax. Metronidazole and gentamicin are given at the time of surgery. The haemoglobin is checked and blood transfusion is given if necessary.

Operative

The principle of operative treatment is wide resection of the tumour together with its regional lymph nodes. This achieves cure in 75% of intended curative resections.

In the unobstructed case, the bowel can be prepared beforehand and primary resection with restoration of continuity can be achieved. In the obstructed case, where bowel preparation is contraindicated, the primary goal is to relieve obstruction.

Typical operations in colorectal cancer

Location of cancer	Operation
Right/transverse	Right/extended right hemicolectomy
Left	Left hemicolectomy
Sigmoid/upper rectum	High anterior resection
Anorectal	Abdomino-perineal resection (APER)
Lower rectum	Low anterior resection/APER

Chemoradiotherapy

Preoperative (neoadjuvant) chemoradio-
therapy may be used in rectal cancer
to increase the chance of curative
resection. Furthermore, systemic adjuvant
chemotherapy using 5-FU alone or in
combination has been shown to improve
survival for Duke's stage C colorectal cancer
after surgical resection, with an overall 30%
improvement in survival.

Palliative treatment may be needed for
unresectable metastases or unresectable
tumours.

Resources

SIGN *Diagnosis and management of colorectal cancer,
Guideline 126* (2016): www.sign.ac.uk/assets/
sign126.pdf

Case 12: Acute loin pain and haematuria

Presenting complaint

▸ SE is a 26-year-old gentleman with known renal stone disease who presented with acute loin pain and frank haematuria.

History of presenting complaint

▸ SE presented to accident and emergency with a 2-day history of severe, intermittent right loin pain and one episode of frank haematuria. The pain was stabbing in nature and initially localised to the right flank.

▸ However, over the 2 days prior to admission, the pain intensified and radiated to the bladder. He also passed a large amount of blood-red urine which prompted him to seek medical attention.

▸ He experienced other urinary symptoms including frequency, hesitancy and dysuria.

▸ He felt generally unwell, was very nauseous and vomited.

Past medical history

▸ SE has known urinary tract stone disease. He was admitted 2 years ago with a similar problem. He was unsure of what treatment he received.

▸ Depression.

Drug history

Drug	Class	Dose	Frequency	Indication
Citalopram	SSRI	20 mg	od	Depression

Allergies

▸ NKDA.

Family history

▸ No significant family history. Both his parents are still alive and he does not think that they have any illness or urological disease.

▸ He has a brother (22) and a sister (29). Both are well.

Social history

▶ SE has been in a relationship with his girlfriend for 6 years.

▶ He works as a ski instructor.

▶ He smokes 6–8 cigarettes a day and says that he is a 'social' drinker and will only drink on special occasions. He admitted to smoking two cannabis joints a week.

Systemic enquiry

▶ **Neurological:** No falls, LOC, seizures or dizziness. Occasional headaches.

▶ **Cardiovascular:** No ankle oedema or chest pain.

▶ **Respiratory:** No dyspnoea, orthopnoea, PND.

▶ **Genitourinary:** Frank haematuria; dysuria; hesitancy; frequency. No nocturia or incontinence.

▶ **Gastrointestinal:** No change in bowel habit. No melaena. Generalised abdominal pain. Nausea and vomiting. Poor appetite.

▶ **Musculoskeletal:** Nil.

Physical examination

General

▶ SG is in bed and looks unwell. He is pale and sweaty.

Vital signs

▶ Temp 38.1°C

▶ RR 20 breaths/minute

▶ BP 130/100 mmHg

▶ O_2 sats 100% on air.

▶ HR 110 bpm – regular

Cardiovascular

▶ No visible JVP

▶ Apex beat in fifth intercostal space in the mid-clavicular line

▶ S1, S2; regular rate

▶ Peripheral pulses present

▶ No oedema.

Respiratory

▶ Chest clear.

▶ No added sounds or wheeze.

Gastrointestinal/abdominal

▶ No scars, spider naevi, gynaecomastia, jaundice or hepatic flap

▶ Tender in the LIF and suprapubic region

▶ No organomegaly

▶ Bowel sounds active.

≣ Summary of patient's problems

▶ Severe loin pain

▶ Haematuria.

❷ Questions

▶ Based on the patient's symptoms, what are the main differential diagnoses?

▶ What initial investigations would help confirm the diagnosis?

▶ What is your immediate management plan?

Differential diagnosis

- Urinary calculi
- UTI
- Appendicitis
- Cholecystitis
- Diverticulitis
- Pyelonephritis.

Initial management plan

- Assess ABCDE
- Establish IV access
- Request bloods (FBC, U+Es, LFTs, CRP, amylase)
- IV fluids
- Analgesia (diclofenac 100 mg PR – best for renal colic)
- Antiemetic (metoclopramide 10 mg IV)
- Paracetamol for temperature
- X-ray kidney, ureters and bladder (KUB) or if able immediate CT KUB
- NBM.

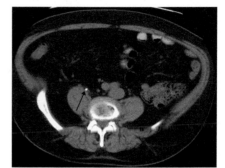

Results of investigations

- **Bloods** were unremarkable
- **Urinalysis** showed presence of blood and protein
- **CT KUB** revealed the presence of a stone (<0.5 cm) in the right lower ureter (stone shows up as white because of calcium content).

Diagnosis

- Renal colic

SE is a 26-year-old male who presented to accident and emergency with a 2-day history of severe, acute, intermittent right loin pain and one episode of frank haematuria. A CT KUB confirmed the diagnosis of renal calculi.

Management plan

- Continue analgesia
- Monitor fluid balance
- Encourage hydration
- Wait for stone to pass expectantly due to size, but if pain continues intervention may be required.

Background information: renal calculi

In the UK, the prevalence of stones in the population is around 3%. Most stones occur in the upper urinary tract; the incidence of bladder stones has declined in the UK, but in some developing countries they are still common.

Most stones are composed of calcium oxalate and phosphate; these are more common in men by 2:1. Mixed infective stones, which account for about 15% of all calculi, are twice as common in women as in men. The overall male-to-female ratio of stone disease is 2:1.

More than 50% of patients with a history of nephrolithiasis will have a recurrence within 10 years. The risk of recurrence increases if a metabolic or other abnormality predisposing to stone formation is present and is not modified by treatment.

Causes

▶ Dehydration

▶ Infection

▶ Hypercalcaemia

▶ Cystinuria

▶ Renal tubular acidosis

▶ Hypercalciuria

▶ Primary renal disease (e.g. polycystic kidneys)

▶ Drugs.

If the glomerular filtration rate (GFR) is normal, hypercalcaemia almost invariably leads to hypercalciuria. The common causes of hypercalcaemia leading to stone formation are:

▶ primary hyperparathyroidism

▶ vitamin D ingestion

▶ sarcoidosis.

Hypercalciuria

Approximately 8% of men excrete in excess of 7.5 mmol of calcium in 24 hours. Calcium stone formation is more common in this group, but as the majority of even these individuals do not form stones the definition of 'pathological' hypercalciuria is arbitrary. A reasonable definition is 24-hour calcium excretion of more than 7.5 mmol in male stone-formers and more than 6.25 mmol in female stone-formers.

The kidney is the major site for plasma calcium regulation. Approximately 90% of the ionised calcium filtered by the kidney is reabsorbed. Renal tubular reabsorption is controlled largely by parathyroid hormone (PTH).

Approximately 65% of the filtered calcium is absorbed in the proximal convoluted tubule, 20% by the thick ascending limb of the loop of Henle, and 15% by the distal convoluted tubule and collecting ducts.

Causes of hypercalciuria are:

▶ hypercalcaemia

▶ an excessive dietary intake of calcium

▶ excessive resorption of calcium from the skeleton, such as occurs with prolonged immobilisation

▶ idiopathic hypercalciuria.

Idiopathic hypercalciuria is a common risk factor for the formation of stones, and uncontrolled hypercalciuria is a cause of recurrences. The majority of patients with idiopathic hypercalciuria have increased absorption of calcium from the gut.

Dehydration alone may also cause uric acid stones to form. Patients with ileostomies are at particular risk both from dehydration and from the fact that loss of bicarbonate from GI secretions results in the production of acidic urine (uric acid is more soluble in an alkaline than in an acid medium).

UTIs

Mixed infective stones are composed of magnesium ammonium phosphate together with variable amounts of calcium. Such struvite stones are often large, forming a cast of the collecting system (staghorn calculus).

Staghorn calculi fill the calcyceal system. These stones are usually due to UTI with organisms such as *Proteus mirabilis* that hydrolyse urea, with formation of the strong base ammonium hydroxide. The availability of ammonium ions and the alkalinity of the urine favour stone formation. An increased production of mucoprotein from infection also creates an organic matrix on which stone formation can occur.

Primary renal disease

There is a high prevalence of stone disease in patients with polycystic renal disease.

Medullary sponge kidney is also associated with stones. There is dilatation of the collecting ducts with associated stasis and calcification. Approximately 20% of these patients have hypercalciuria and a similar proportion have a renal tubular acidification defect.

Renal tubular acidosis, whether inherited or acquired, is associated with nephrocalcinosis and stone formation, owing, in part, to the production of persistently alkaline urine and reduced urinary citrate excretion.

Drugs

Some drugs promote calcium stone formation (e.g. loop diuretics, antacids, glucocorticoids, theophylline, vitamins D and C, acetazolamide); some promote uric acid stones (e.g. thiazides, salicylates); and some precipitate into stones (e.g. indinavir).

Clinical features

▸ Ureteric/renal colic – severe, intermittent, stabbing pain radiating from the loin to the groin

▸ Microscopic, or rarely, frank haematuria

▸ Systemic symptoms such as nausea, vomiting, tachycardia and pyrexia

▸ Loin or renal angle tenderness due to infection or inflammation

▸ Iliac fossa tenderness if the calculus has passed into the distal ureter.

Renal colic

Renal colic usually begins in the upper lateral mid back over the costovertebral angle and occasionally subcostally. The pain generated by renal colic is primarily caused by the dilation, stretching and spasm caused by the acute ureteric obstruction. A stone lodged at the neck of a calyx or at the pelvi-ureteric junction causes waves of increasing pain often superimposed on a background of continuous nagging pain at the same site. The pain radiates inferiorly and anteriorly toward the groin.

Investigations

These should include a mid-stream specimen of urine for culture and measurement of serum urea, electrolyte, creatinine and calcium levels.

Imaging

▸ A KUB is a plain film of the abdomen. Approximately 85% of kidney stones can be identified with the KUB, as the calcium component present in most kidney stones can be seen on the KUB. Only uric acid is truly radiolucent.

▸ This quick, inexpensive X-ray can often tell the size and number of stones present.

▸ Non-contrast spiral CT is the gold standard for locating stones and assessing evidence of complications.

▸ Intravenous urogram (IVU) will locate stones and show any proximal obstruction.

▸ Renal ultrasound scan to identify hydronephrosis.

Treatment

Acute presentations

▶ Ensure adequate analgesia

▶ An NSAID, e.g. diclofenac 100 mg PR

▶ Metoclopramide 10 mg IV

▶ Give IV fluids if patient is unable to tolerate orally

▶ Stones less than 0.5 cm diameter usually pass spontaneously – patients are advised to increase fluid intake and sieve the urine to catch the stone for biochemical analysis; their progress can be monitored on serial abdominal films every 1–2 weeks

▶ Emergency treatment with percutaneous nephrostomy and/or ureteric stent insertion is necessary if either pain or obstruction persist.

Elective presentations

Stones greater than 1 cm usually require urological or radiological intervention.

▶ Extracorporeal shock wave lithotripsy (ESWL) – focused, externally generated electrohydraulic or ultrasonic shock waves are targeted on the calculus to cause stone disintegration and the fragments are then voided.

▶ Percutaneous nephrolithotomy – for stones in the renal pelvis or calyces. Percutaneous track into the renal pelvis using fluoroscopic guidance. Nephroscope is inserted and the calculus visualised and removed.

▶ Endoscopic treatment – ureteroscope is inserted and stone visualised. Stone is fragmented using ultrasound, electrohydraulic intracorporeal lithotripsy, or laser.

▶ Open surgery is rarely needed.

Prevention

▶ Patients are advised to drink plenty of fluid, especially in summer or warm weather (aim for 2–3 L a day of colourless urine).

▶ A normal calcium intake is recommended, as low calcium diets increase oxalate excretion.

Specifically:

▶ **Calcium stones** – if there is hypercalciuria, a thiazide diuretic (e.g. bendroflumethiazide) is used to decrease calcium excretion.

▶ **Oxalate stones** – oxalate intake is reduced (less tea, chocolate, nuts, strawberries, rhubarb, spinach, beans and beetroot). Pyridoxine may be used.

▶ **Magnesium ammonium phosphate** – treat infection promptly.

▶ **Urate stones** – allopurinol (100–300 mg/ 24 h PO) to decrease uric acid. Urine alkalisation may also be recommended, as urate is more soluble at pH >6 (e.g. with potassium citrate or sodium bicarbonate).

▶ **Cystine stones:** Vigorous hydration to keep urine output >3 L a day and urinary alkalisation. D-penicillamine is used to chelate cystine, given with pyridoxine to prevent vitamin B6 deficiency.

Resources

NICE *Renal and ureteric stones: assessment and management, NG118* (2019): www.nice.org.uk/ guidance/ng118

Case 13:   Left iliac fossa pain

Presenting complaint

▶ MD is a 55-year-old lady who presented with pain in her left iliac fossa (LIF) and a 3-day history of diarrhoea.

History of presenting complaint

▶ MD presented to her GP with a 3-day history of abdominal pain and diarrhoea. The pain was initially in the epigastric region, but went on to localise in the LIF and suprapubic region.

▶ She describes the pain as severe, sharp and constant. It is aggravated by movement.

▶ The pain was followed by the onset of 'explosive' diarrhoea, which she has had for the past two days. She also experienced pain after defecation. She is unaware of any PR bleeding, melaena or mucus.

▶ The pain and diarrhoea are accompanied by nausea, but she has not vomited. Her appetite is also very poor.

▶ She also complains of dysuria and says that her urine has been a cloudy, white colour for the past 2 days. She has also experienced hesitancy and frequency. She is not aware of any frank haematuria.

Past medical history

▶ Known diverticular disease, diagnosed 5 years ago; her last admission for diverticular disease was 2 years ago

▶ Irritable bowel syndrome (IBS)

▶ Low back pain

▶ Hysterectomy and right oophorectomy (20 years ago for menorrhagia and cystic disease, respectively).

Drug history

▶ Nil.

Allergies

▶ NKDA.

Family history

▶ MD's father died from ischaemic heart disease at the age of 51.

▶ Her mother is 81 years old and has rheumatoid arthritis.

▶ She has a sister (50) and a brother (48) who are both well.

Social history

▶ MD previously owned a pub but had to give this up due to the onset of low back pain.

▶ She now works as a training consultant and is self-employed.

▶ She has been married twice. Her first marriage ended in 2000 and she had four children in this relationship (aged 36, 32, 23, and 21).

▶ She re-married in 2003, but unfortunately this was an abusive relationship and ended this year. MD is now living in a women's refuge for those affected by domestic abuse.

▶ She is a non-smoker and only drinks occasionally as she feels that alcohol has a negative impact on her diverticular disease.

Systemic enquiry

▶ **Neurological:** Occasional headaches; no LOC, faints, seizures or dizziness; no paraesthesia or muscle weakness.

▶ **Cardiovascular:** No ankle oedema or chest pain; no SOB.

▶ **Respiratory:** No cough or wheeze; no haemoptysis or sputum; no dyspnoea, orthopnoea or PND.

▶ **Genitourinary:** Dysuria, frequency and hesitancy.

▶ **Gastrointestinal:** 'explosive' diarrhoea; no PR bleeding, melaena or mucus. Generalised abdominal pain that is worse in the LIF and suprapubic region.

▶ **Musculoskeletal:** Nil.

Physical examination

General

▶ MD is lying comfortably reading in bed.

Vital signs

▶ Temp 36.2°C
▶ BP 110/80 mmHg
▶ HR 85 bpm – regular
▶ RR 16 breaths/minute
▶ O₂ sats 97% on air.

Cardiovascular

▶ No visible JVP

▶ Apex beat in the fifth intercostal space in the mid-clavicular line

▶ S1, S2; regular rate

▶ Peripheral pulses present

▶ No oedema.

Respiratory

▶ Chest clear

▶ No added sounds.

Gastrointestinal/abdominal

▶ No hepatic flap, jaundice or signs of anaemia

▶ Old McBurney scar and a large lower abdominal midline scar

▶ The abdomen was soft; generally globally tender on palpation but more so in the LIF and suprapubic region

▶ No guarding or rebound tenderness

▶ No organomegaly

▶ Hyperactive bowel sounds.

☰ Summary of patient's problems

▶ Left iliac fossa pain

▶ Diarrhoea.

---

❷ Questions

▶ Based on the patient's symptoms, what are the main differential diagnoses?

▶ What initial investigations would help confirm the diagnosis?

▶ What is your immediate management plan?

Differential diagnosis

▸ Acute diverticulitis

▸ UTI

▸ IBS

▸ Left tubo-ovarian pathology (e.g. ovarian cyst, infection, torsion, etc).

Initial management plan

▸ Assess ABCDE

▸ IV access

▸ Request bloods (FBC, U+Es, LFTs, CRP and glucose)

▸ IV fluids

▸ Analgesia and antiemetic (Buscopan, cyclizine, co-codamol/morphine)

▸ Urinalysis

▸ CT abdomen.

Results of investigations

Blood results

Substance	Reference range	Result
Na^+	135–145 mmol/L	141 mmol/L
K^+	3.5–5.0 mmol/L	3.9 mmol/L
Cl^-	97–107 mmol/L	106 mmol/L
HCO_3^-	23–30 mmol/L	26 mmol/L
Urea	2.5–6.7 mmol/L	5.3 mmol/L
Creatinine	40–130 µmol/L	7.5 µmol/L
ALT	3–35 U/L	53 U/L
AST	3–35 U/L	38 U/L
Alk phos	40–150 U/L	99 U/L
Hb	115–165 g/L	138 g/L
WCC	$4–11 \times 10^9$/L	5.4×10^9/L
CRP	<10 mg/L	150 mg/L
Glucose	3.5–6.0 mmol/L	5.3 mmol/L

Urinalysis

▸ Positive for blood, leuk ++, trace protein.

Other

▸ MD was commenced on trimethoprim for presumed UTI. However, the following day she had increasing left iliac pain and she was commenced on IV antibiotics.

CT abdo

▸ CT abdomen confirmed acute diverticulitis.

Diagnosis

▸ Acute diverticulitis

MD, a 55-year-old lady with known diverticular disease, presented with a 3-day history of pain in the left iliac fossa and suprapubic region. The pain was severe, sharp and constant. The abdomen was generally globally tender on palpation but more so in the LIF. CT confirmed diverticulitis.

Further management plan

▸ Continue IV fluids

▸ Continue analgesia

▸ IV antibiotics (local guidelines).

Background information: diverticular disease

A diverticulum is an outpouching of part or all of a viscus. Diverticular disease of the colon is very rarely congenital, in which case the walls of the diverticula contain all the layers of the normal colon. Much more commonly it is acquired and the diverticula are serosa-covered outpouchings of mucosa alone through gaps in the muscularis which transmit the terminal blood vessels. The diverticula are usually found in the left colon, especially the sigmoid, but can involve the entire colon.

Epidemiology

Acquired diverticular disease is very rare under the age of 35, after which there is a progressive increase in incidence. It is common in Western countries but rare in China, India and Africa.

Aetiology

It is thought that a diet low in fibre is associated with increased intraluminal pressure which results in herniation of the mucosa through the muscle coats of the colonic wall. Diverticula tend to occur along the lines where penetrating colonic arteries traverse the colonic wall between the taenia coli.

Clinical and pathological features

Asymptomatic

The majority of diverticular disease is found incidentally on barium enema examination.

Painful diverticular disease

Intermittent LIF pain may be due to diverticular disease, but IBS commonly coexists and may be the cause of the symptoms.

Acute diverticulitis

Rapid onset of LIF pain, nausea, fever, frequently with loose stools. Usually febrile with moderate tachycardia and left iliac tenderness. Frequency and haematuria are the result of adherence of the inflamed loop of colon to the bladder.

Biopsy of the colonic wall shows acute neutrophil infiltration around the inflamed diverticulum and in the subserosal tissues.

The diagnosis is primarily a clinical one, with the typical presentation being sufficient to treat the patient expectantly. Treatment comprises:

- Clear fluids by mouth
- Bed rest
- IV fluids
- Broad-spectrum antibiotic (cephalosporin or metronidazole).

Failure to settle suggests the development of pericolic abscess, and surgery may be required. In the absence of rapid improvement within 36–48 hours, intravenous and oral contrast CT should be undertaken. Approximately 1/3 of all patients admitted with acute diverticular disease undergo surgery, while the remainder settle and have no further attacks. Around 10% of these patients will eventually require surgery comprising sigmoid colectomy with primary anastomosis.

Bleeding diverticular disease

Usually spontaneous in onset with no prodromal symptoms. Presenting with large volume, dark red, clotted rectal blood. Due to rupture of a peridiverticular submucosal blood vessel. It is not usually associated with inflammation.

Complicated diverticular disease

Pericolic/paracolic mass/abscess

Acute diverticulitis may progress to persistent pericolic infection with thickening of surrounding tissues and the formation of a mass. If this suppurates, a pericolic abscess forms. Enlargement and extension into the paracolic area leads to a paracolic abscess.

The features are those of acute diverticulitis with a swinging fever, fluctuating tachycardia, unresolving abdominal pain, and a tender LIF mass.

Peritonitis

Perforation of a pericolic or paracolic abscess usually leads to purulent peritonitis. Direct perforation of the acute diverticular segment leads to faeculent peritonitis. The features are those of acute diverticulitis with high fever, severe abdominal pain, and generalised guarding and rigidity.

Diverticular fistula

Acute infection with paracolic sepsis may drain by perforation into adjacent structures. This is typically the posterior vaginal vault in women or the bladder in either sex. Colovesical fistula leads to recurrent UTI caused by enteric organisms, with bubbles and debris in the urine. Colovaginal fistula leads to faeculent vaginal discharge.

Stricture formation

Chronic and repetitive inflammatory episodes may lead to fibrosis and narrowing of the colon. A history of recurrent diverticulitis with recurrent colicky abdominal pain, distension and bloating suggests stricture formation.

Diagnosis and investigations

▶ Elective diagnosis is usually by double contrast barium enema

▶ Colonoscopy is relatively poor at assessing the number and extent of diverticula

▶ Hb, WCC, CRP during acute episodes

▶ CT is the best investigation to assess complications

▶ Colonoscopy is indicated if there is any suggestion of coexistent malignancy.

Treatment

Medical

▶ A high-fibre diet, high fluid intake and stool softeners are used to reduce intracolonic pressure

▶ IV antibiotics during acute exacerbations

▶ Recurrent infective episodes may be prevented by a 6-week course of oral antibiotics (e.g. ciprofloxacin 500 mg PO)

▶ Significant paracolic abscesses may be drained by radiological guidance.

Surgical

▶ Resection is indicated for: acute inflammation failing to respond to medical management; undrainable paracolic sepsis; or free perforation; the affected region should be resected (segmental colectomy)

▶ Stricture may be treated by elective resection or intracolonic stenting

▶ Diverticular fistula should be treated by elective resection to prevent recurrent infections.

Resources

NICE *Diverticular disease: diagnosis and management, GID-NG10064* (2019): www.nice.org.uk/guidance/gid-ng10064

Case 14: Abdominal pain and jaundice

👤 Presenting complaint

▶ JK is a 55-year-old architect who presented with a 6-week history of lower abdominal pain and a 4-week history of jaundice.

History of presenting complaint

▶ Six weeks ago, JK experienced the gradual onset of generalised lower abdominal pain. The pain is colicky, severe and associated with nausea. It does not radiate. It is aggravated by movement, coughing and swallowing, and is partially relieved by painkillers.

▶ Two weeks after the onset of pain, JK noticed a yellow discolouration of his skin and sclera. He also had dark urine and pale stools.

▶ There was no other change in bowel habit, no melaena or PR bleeding.

▶ He has lost 1.5 stone (9.5 kg) in weight over 6 weeks. His appetite is also very poor and he says that he 'gags' after food.

▶ Steatorrhoea.

▶ No pruritus.

▶ No fever.

▶ He has not been on holiday recently, does not drink alcohol and has never taken IV drugs.

Past medical history

▶ 20-year history of ulcerative colitis: he has not been affected by this in the last 5 years; it has always been well controlled medically and has never required surgery

▶ Depression/anxiety   ▶ No previous operations.

Drug history

Drug	Class	Dose	Frequency	Indication
Azathioprine	Immunosuppressant (interferes with purine synthesis)	75 mg	od	Inflammatory bowel disease
Fluoxetine	SSRI	10 mg	od	Depression
Omeprazole	PPI	20 mg	od	Gastric protection

Allergies

▶ NKDA.

Family history

▶ Mother died aged 78 from lung cancer.

▶ Father died aged 41 from 'blood disorder'.

▶ JK had two brothers who are now deceased. One died at the age of 61 as a result of emphysema. The other died at the age of 60 after choking.

▶ He has one remaining brother, who has bipolar disorder.

Social history

▶ JK has been married to his wife for 21 years. They live in a three-bedroom, top-floor flat. They don't have any children.

▶ His wife works from home, as she is a writer. He is an architect.

▶ JK has not drunk alcohol in the last 2–3 years. He attributes this to his depression, which was worsened by alcohol. Previous to this, he says he occasionally binged on alcohol.

▶ He is an ex-smoker, having quit 5 years ago. He says he was a 'light' smoker before giving up.

▶ He smoked cannabis recreationally in the past. No other recreational drug use.

Systemic enquiry

▶ **Neurological:** Nil.

▶ **Cardiovascular:** Nil.

▶ **Respiratory:** Nil.

▶ **Genitourinary:** Dark urine.

▶ **Gastrointestinal:** Abdominal pain; nausea; yellow discolouration of skin and sclera; weight loss; decreased appetite.

▶ **Musculoskeletal:** Nil.

Physical examination

General

▶ Alert gentleman who is lying in bed. He is clearly jaundiced and appears rather lethargic. He looks underweight.

Vital signs

▶ HR 64 bpm – regular

▶ BP 130/75 mmHg

▶ RR 16 breaths/minute

▶ O_2 sats 97% on air.

Cardiovascular

- No visible JVP
- S1, S2; regular rate
- No oedema
- Apex beat in fifth intercostal space in the mid-clavicular line
- Peripheral pulses present
- No murmurs.

Respiratory

- No use of accessory muscles
- Equal air entry
- Thorax symmetrical; good expansion
- No added sounds.

Gastrointestinal/abdominal

- No finger clubbing, Dupuytren's contractures, palmar erythema or koilonychia
- Jaundice
- No gynaecomastia, spider naevi
- Troisier's sign (negative)
- The abdomen is hard but not distended; no abdominal scars
- Bowel sounds active
- No guarding or rebound tenderness
- No obvious masses
- Tender on palpation in the lower abdomen
- No hernias.

≔ Summary of patient's problems

- Jaundice
- Nausea
- Abdominal pain
- Poor appetite and weight loss.

❓ Questions

- Based on the patient's symptoms, what are the main differential diagnoses?
- What initial investigations would help confirm the diagnosis?
- What is your immediate management plan?

Differential diagnosis

▸ Pancreatitis

▸ Hepatitis

▸ Gallstones

▸ Sclerosing cholangitis

▸ Cholangiocarcinoma

▸ Tumours, e.g. head of pancreas, ampulla of Vater.

Management plan

▸ Assess ABCDE

▸ IV access and bloods

▸ IV fluids

▸ Consider urinary catheter; monitor hourly urine output

▸ Analgesia and antiemetic

▸ Bloods (FBC, U+Es, LFTs, amylase, CRP)

▸ Abdominal ultrasound

▸ Endoscopic retrograde cholangiopancreatography (ERCP).

Results of investigations

Blood results

Substance	Reference range	Result
Na$^+$	135–145 mmol/L	138 mmol/L
K$^+$	3.5–5.0 mmol/L	4.3 mmol/L
Urea	2.5–6.7 mmol/L	4.1 mmol/L
Creatinine	70–150 µmol/L	94 µmol/L
Ca^{2+}	2.12–2.65 mmol/L	2.34 mmol/L
Bilirubin	3–17 µmol/L	380 µmol/L
ALT	3–35 U/L	161 U/L
AST	3–35 U/L	151 U/L
Gamma-GT	11–51 U/L	1551 U/L
Amylase	<100 U/L	3900 U/L
Hb	130–180 g/L	132 g/L

(continued overleaf)

Substance	Reference range	Result
WCC	4–11 × 10⁹/L	7 × 10⁹/L
Platelets	150–400 × 10⁹/L	429 × 10⁹/L
CRP	<10 mg/L	38 mg/L

❓ Question

▸ What type of jaundice are the blood tests indicative of?

Abdominal ultrasound

▸ Dilated common bile duct (1.2 cm)

▸ No focal liver lesion and no obvious pancreatic mass was identified.

ERCP

Cannulation via major papilla to the bile and pancreatic ducts.

▸ Ampulla and pancreas normal

▸ Biliary stricture – probably malignant, length 2 cm, irregular and with upstream dilatation

▸ Biliary extrahepatic stricture – malignant – probably cholangiocarcinoma.

Diagnosis

▸ Cholangiocarcinoma complicated by post-ERCP pancreatitis

JK is a 55-year-old architect who presented with a 6-week history of abdominal pain and jaundice. His urine is dark, his stools are pale and he has lost 1.5 stone (9.5 kg) in the past 6 weeks. He has a long-standing history of ulcerative colitis. Investigations revealed grossly abnormal obstructive LFTs and elevated CRP. An abdominal ultrasound revealed a dilated common bile duct, and ERCP indicated extrahepatic malignancy.

Further management

Management will involve supportive measures and CT to determine the extent of disease.

Background information: pancreatitis

Pancreatitis is an inflammatory disorder of the pancreas that is characterised by abdominal pain. Pancreatitis may be acute or chronic.

The incidence of acute pancreatitis in the UK appears to be rising, with approximately 56 cases per 100 000 people per year. Pancreatic injury results in an inflammatory process with the cascade of inflammatory cytokines, such as tumour necrosis factor (TNF)-α, interleukin (IL)-2, IL-6, and platelet-activating factor (PAF). In addition pancreatic enzymes including trypsin, lipases and co-lipases are released.

There are many causes of acute pancreatitis, but alcohol and gallstones are thought to be the causal factor in 80% of cases worldwide.

Causes

▶ Gallstones (60%)

▶ Alcohol (30%)

▶ Hyperlipidaemia

▶ Idiopathic

▶ Direct damage (trauma, ERCP, after surgery, cardiopulmonary bypass)

▶ Toxic

> drugs, e.g. azathioprine, oestrogens, thiazides, isoniazid, steroids

> infection, e.g. viral (mumps, cytomegalovirus, hepatitis B), mycoplasma

> venom (scorpion sting, snake bites).

Gallstones

Gallstones are rarely associated with chronic pancreatitis but are often associated with recurrent acute attacks unless they are surgically removed. The exact mechanism by which gallstones cause acute pancreatitis is not fully understood. However, patients with numerous small stones are more likely to develop acute pancreatitis than those with large solitary stones. It is now thought that stones may impact transiently in the major papilla and so promote reflux of bile or duodenal contents into the pancreatic duct. Reflux leads to the activation of pro-enzymes which destroy cell membranes, ultimately causing autodigestion of the pancreas, and the development of oedema, vascular damage and necrosis.

Alcohol

Like gallstones, the precise mechanism by which alcohol leads to damage is unknown. However, alcohol has a toxic effect on the pancreas, and excessive drinking can precipitate an acute episode of pancreatitis. It has been postulated that alcohol consumption may lead to the secretion of unusually viscid juice which contributes to the occurrence of protein plugs that impair flow and may also generate toxic free radicals.

Classification/complications

Oedematous pancreatitis

This milder form of pancreatitis makes up 70% of cases. It is characterised by interstitial oedema with inflammatory exudate.

Severe/necrotising

Glandular necrosis occurs in this more severe form in 25% of acute pancreatitis cases. Necrotising pancreatitis results from microcirculatory stasis within the pancreas leading to infarction. The necrosis may be sterile or infected, and persistent pseudocysts containing large amounts of peripancreatic fluid may form. These too may become infected.

Clinical features

The principal symptom is abdominal pain, from mild discomfort to excruciating in severe cases. The pain is usually localised to the epigastrium or upper abdomen, but may radiate to the upper lumbar region between the scapulae.

Most cases are accompanied by nausea and vomiting. Fever, dehydration, hypotension and tachycardia (shock in severe cases) may occur too.

Epigastric tenderness is common, associated with guarding and, in severe cases, rigidity.

Rarely, haemorrhagic tracking from the retroperitoneum results in body wall ecchymoses around the umbilicus (Cullen's sign) or in the flanks (Grey Turner's sign).

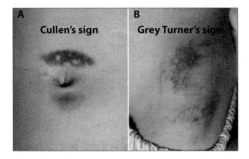

Diagnosis

The diagnosis of acute pancreatitis may be difficult to make despite the many types of investigation available. It is imperative that other life-threatening conditions are excluded (for example, mesenteric ischaemia, visceral perforation, leaking AAA).

Clinical

Common clinical findings such as a history of upper abdominal pain and vomiting with features of epigastric or diffuse abdominal pain should raise suspicion.

Biochemical

Elevation of serum amylase occurs in a number of acute abdominal emergencies including acute cholecystitis, bowel ischaemia and perforated peptic ulcer, but a concentration in excess of 1000 U/L (or four times the upper limit of normal) is highly suggestive of acute pancreatitis.

Radiology

Chest and abdominal plain X-ray examinations should be performed routinely to provide a baseline picture and to exclude other pathology such as perforated viscus and intestinal obstruction.

The reported plain abdominal X-ray findings in acute pancreatitis are non-specific. They include: absent psoas shadows; 'sentinel loop sign' (dilated proximal jejunal loop adjacent to pancreas because of local ileus); 'colon cut-off sign' (distended colon to mid-transverse colon with no air distally); gallstones or pancreatic calcification may be visible. These appearances are non-specific and cannot be recommended for use in diagnosis. Rarely, in advanced cases, the presence of retroperitoneal gas will indicate infection.

Ultrasound

Ultrasound examination of the abdomen may be helpful in confirming the diagnosis. A swollen pancreas may be detected. Ultrasound is valuable in detecting free peritoneal fluid, gallstones, dilatation of the common bile duct, and occasionally other pathology such as AAA.

Computed tomography

A CT may be required if the diagnosis is uncertain. This would illustrate pancreatic oedema, swelling and loss of fat planes, and may show haemorrhagic complications.

Prognosis

The severity of an attack can be assessed in a number of ways. This will be influenced by the clinical condition of the patient, prognostic factor measurements (CRP), and by prognostic factor scoring systems.

The Glasgow Imrie criteria are widely used to determine severity. Three or more positive criteria (one point each) within 48 hours of admission relates to a severe attack.

Glasgow Imrie criteria
Age >55 years
WCC >15000 × 10⁹/L
Glucose >7 mmol/L
Blood urea >7 mmol/L
Albumin <35 g/L
Corrected Ca²⁺ <2 mmol/L
PaO_2 <10 kPa

Management

No specific treatment is available and management is thus supportive. Mild pancreatitis usually resolves with parenteral fluid replacement, bowel rest (NBM) and analgesia.

A severe attack needs more intensive therapy and should ideally be managed in the high-dependency unit (HDU):

▸ IV antibiotics as per local guidelines.

▸ HDU/ITU – optimised fluid balance, respiratory, cardiovascular and renal support.

▸ For proven infected necrosis, surgical debridement may be required, but it is associated with poor prognosis.

Resources

NICE *Pancreatitis: diagnosis and management NG104* (2018): www.nice.org.uk/guidance/ng104

Case 15: Necrotic foot

👤 Presenting complaint

▸ JR is a 50-year-old man with type 1 diabetes who presented with a necrotic left foot.

History of presenting complaint

▸ 18 months ago JR noticed that he had two small lacerations on the heel of his left foot. These failed to heal and JR said that he noticed 'black marks' on the sole of his left foot. He did not experience any pain.

▸ He then went to his GP who subsequently referred him to hospital.

▸ His left foot was extensively affected by dry necrosis. The entire forefoot was irretrievably ischaemic and there was also a large patch of necrosis on the lateral aspect of the heel. There was a penetrating ulcer on the sole of his right foot.

▸ JR said that after ten days in hospital the necrosis had spread to the level of his left ankle. Despite the extent of necrosis, JR was not keen to have surgery. He was discharged and did not seek further medical attention for over a year.

▸ Three weeks ago, JR was admitted for a below-knee amputation. He has subsequently had his operation and has been getting regular physiotherapy. Since the procedure, he has experienced episodes of pain in his stump which mostly occur at night.

▸ The wound is failing to heal sufficiently and he remains an inpatient for wound care.

Past medical history

▸ Type 1 diabetes mellitus (20 years)

▸ Hypertension

▸ Amputation in right fifth toe

▸ Renal failure

▸ Non-proliferative diabetic retinopathy.

▸ Stent (left anterior descending artery)

▸ Back pain

▸ Angina

▸ Anaemia

Drug history

Drug	Class	Dose	Frequency	Indication
Paracetamol	COX inhibitor	1 g	od	Pain
NovoRapid	Recombinant human insulin analogue (short-acting)	8 units	Immediately before meals or when necessary shortly after meals	Type 1 diabetes mellitus

Drug	Class	Dose	Frequency	Indication
Lantus	insulin (long-acting)	3 units	At bedtime	Type 1 diabetes mellitus
Ferrous fumarate	Iron supplement	210 mg	bd	Iron-deficiency anaemia
Lansoprazole	PPI	15 mg	od	Dyspepsia
Allopurinol	Xanthine oxidase inhibitor	100 mg	od	Prophylaxis of gout
Nicorandil	Potassium-channel activator	20 mg	bd	Angina
Ezetimibe	Cholesterol absorption inhibitor	10 mg	od	Hypercholesterolaemia
Bisoprolol	Beta-blocker	5 mg	od	Angina
Augmentin	Co-amoxiclav	250 mg	tds	Infection prophylaxis

Allergies

▶ NKDA.

Family history

▶ JR's father died at the age of 59 due to 'cancer'

▶ His mother (75) is still alive and he says that she is well

▶ He has two sisters (54, 44) and one brother (49). They are all well and JR says that there is no family history of diabetes mellitus.

Social history

▶ JR lives with his mother, and always has

▶ The house has three bedrooms upstairs, which has resulted in some difficulty for JR: even before his amputation, he would have to sit on the stairs and struggle up on his behind

▶ His brother is in the process of arranging an extension to be built on the lower level of the house

▶ JR previously worked as a painter, but his deteriorating health forced him to stop

▶ He has never smoked

▶ He says that he previously 'enjoyed a drink' and would spend most days in the pub; he claims to have cut down considerably over the past couple of years but still drinks around 30 units/week

▶ His diet is poor: he eats very little fruit and vegetables and fries most of his food. He also takes very little exercise.

Systemic enquiry

- **Neurological:** Occasional headaches. No visual disturbance.
- **Cardiovascular:** Exertional chest pain. No SOB.
- **Respiratory:** No cough, haemoptysis or sputum production.
- **Genitourinary:** Polyuria. No nocturia or dysuria.
- **Gastrointestinal:** Constipation. No PR bleeding.
- **Musculoskeletal:** Nil.

Physical examination

General

- Alert, slightly overweight gentleman. There is a wheelchair next to his bed.

Vital signs

- BP 139/72
- HR 100 bpm – regularly
- RR 16 breaths/minute.

Cardiovascular

- No visible JVP
- S1, S2; regular rate
- Apex beat in fifth intercostal space in the mid-clavicular line
- No oedema.

Peripheral vascular system

- JR has a below-the-knee amputation of his left leg
- His right foot is bandaged to the level of the ankle
- Both legs lack hair; his right shin is smooth, shiny, pale and cool to the touch
- Amputated fifth right toe
- The wound on his left leg is failing to heal and there is a 5 cm open wound on the anteromedial aspect of the stump
- There is a penetrating ulcer on the sole of his right foot
- The femoral pulses are reduced bilaterally, though weaker on the left; unable to palpate the popliteal pulse on either side; dorsalis pedis and posterior tibial pulses were absent on the right
- There were no femoral bruits.

≔ Summary of patient's problems

▶ Poorly controlled type 1 diabetes

▶ Penetrating ulcer on the right foot

▶ Postoperative amputation that is slow to heal

▶ Poor mobility

▶ Acute on chronic renal failure.

❓ Questions

▶ Based on the patient's symptoms, what are the main differential diagnoses?

▶ What initial investigations would help confirm the diagnosis?

▶ What is your immediate management plan?

Differential diagnosis

Chronic leg ulcers:

▶ Necrotic foot secondary to poorly controlled diabetes

▶ Vascular (venous, arterial, lymphatic, vasculitis)

▶ Connective tissue disease (IBD, pyoderma gangrenosum, rheumatoid arthritis, scleroderma, systemic lupus erythematosus [SLE], bullous pemphigoid, dermatomyositis, polyarteritis nodosa, leukocytoclastic vasculitis)

▶ Cutaneous microthrombotic ulcers

▶ Neoplasm

▶ Panniculitis

▶ Traumatic (pressure ulcer, radiation damage).

Results of investigations

Blood results

Substance	Reference range	Result
Na$^+$	135–145 mmol/L	133 mmol/L
K$^+$	3.5–5.0 mmol/L	6 mmol/L
Urea	2.5–6.7 mmol/L	23.7 mmol/L
Creatinine	70–150 µmol/L	267 µmol/L
Bilirubin	3–17 µmol/L	4 µmol/L
ALT	3–35 U/L	7 U/L
AST	3–35 U/L	14 U/L
Gamma-GT	11–51 U/L	156 U/L
Alk phos	40–150 U/L	266 U/L
Hb	130–180 g/L	95 g/L
WCC	4–11 × 10^9/L	12.1 × 10^9/L
CRP	<10 mg/L	28 mg/L
PTT	9–13 seconds	27 seconds
INR	2.0–2.5	2.3

PTT, partial thromboplastin time.

Wound swab

Culture: No significant growth.

Diagnosis

▶ Necrotic foot secondary to poorly controlled diabetes

JR is a 50-year-old gentleman with long-standing poorly controlled type 1 diabetes who presented with a necrotic left foot. Management will require wound care, observation of his renal function, and a multidisciplinary approach involving physiotherapists and occupational therapists.

Management plan

▶ Wound care

▶ Continue physiotherapy input

▶ Monitor renal function

▶ OT and dietitian referral.

Background information: the diabetic foot

Foot ulceration, foot infection, foot and limb amputation and some forms of deformity are major forms of disability arising from types 1 and 2 diabetes.

Every year in the UK, 5000 people with diabetes have an amputation – 100 people per week. More than 1 in 10 foot ulcers result in an amputation, meaning people with diabetes are 15 times more likely to undergo major lower limb amputation than non-diabetics. However, it is thought that worldwide around half of all foot ulcers and amputations in people with diabetes are preventable.

People with diabetes mellitus are particularly susceptible to these abnormalities because of other aspects of the disorder, as described below. The ulceration that occurs in diabetic patients is secondary to large vessel or small vessel arterial occlusive disease or neuropathy, or both. Approximately 45% of diabetic foot ulceration has a neuropathic origin; 10% are purely ischaemic; 45% are mixed.

Vascular disease

This develops earlier in life in patients with diabetes and tends to be more severe and distal than in non-diabetics, making intervention more difficult.

Sensory neuropathy

This diminishes protective reactions to minor injuries and to symptoms of ischaemia.

Autonomic neuropathy

A lack of sweating leads to dry, fissured skin, which is at increased risk of infections.

Clinical features

- Ulceration
- Infection
- Sensory neuropathy
- Failure of trivial injuries to heal.

Diagnosis and investigation

In pure neuropathic ulceration the foot may be warm with bounding pulses. It may also be possible to see distended veins and there may be evidence of sensory loss, which can lead to unrecognised repeated local trauma. The duplex ultrasound may show normal or high flow.

When the ulceration is due to ischaemia/neuroischaemia, the foot may be cool to the touch and the pulses may be absent. The ulcers are commonly found on the toes, heel or metatarsal head. Furthermore, secondary infection may be present. When infection is apparent, there is minimal pus and there may be mild surrounding cellulitis. Investigations should include a duplex ultrasound assessment and an angiography for suspected critical ischaemia due to stenosis.

Treatment

Prophylactic management

Management is best undertaken in a multidisciplinary setting. It is imperative that the feet are regularly inspected for signs of pressure/ulceration. The patient should also be advised to:

- wear wide-fitting footwear
- pay attention to nail care, with regular chiropody
- keep away from heat
- not walk barefoot.

Established ischaemic ulceration

Any local or systemic infection must be treated, using broad-spectrum antibiotics (following local guidelines) and the debridement of obviously dead tissue. Pus should be drained and X-rays should be taken for signs of underlying osteomyelitis.

If ischaemic disease is present, re-vascularisation should be considered. This may involve:

▶ angioplasty

▶ femoral distal bypass graft

▶ reconstruction to deal with vascular supply.

If conservative medical or surgical treatment fails, it may be necessary to amputate. The level at which to amputate is chosen according to the lowest level at which tissue is viable for healing and should include as many working joints as possible to improve function.

Lower limb amputations may be:

▶ above knee – most will heal and some achieve walking with a prosthesis

▶ through knee – fewer heal and some achieve walking

▶ below knee – about two-thirds heal and many more achieve walking than with above knee amputations.

Complications of amputations

▶ Infection

▶ Non-healing of stump

▶ Progression of underlying disease requiring higher level amputation

▶ Phantom limb pain due to hypersensitivity of divided nerves (can be helped with gabapentin, amitriptyline or carbamazepine)

▶ Failed mobilisation

▶ Perioperative cardiovascular events in arteriopathic patients.

Resources

NICE *Diabetic foot problems: prevention and management, NG19* (2015): www.nice.org.uk/guidance/ng19

NICE *Diabetic foot infection: antimicrobial prescribing GID-NG10132* (in development): www.nice.org.uk/guidance/GID-NG10132

Case 16: Haematuria

👤 Presenting complaint

▸ MT is an 84-year-old smoker who presented to her GP with painless macroscopic haematuria.

History of presenting complaint

▸ MT noticed that she was passing urine that she describes as the colour of 'cranberry juice'. This occurred in the absence of pain or any other urological symptom such as poor urine flow, hesitancy, frequency, nocturia or incontinence.

▸ MT thought that she had a UTI and did not initially seek medical attention. However, her symptoms persisted for a week and she consulted her GP.

▸ She was subsequently referred for cystoscopy, which showed a bladder lesion.

▸ Transurethral resection of bladder tumour (TURBT) showed a broad-base papillary lesion above the left ureteric orifice and on the left lateral wall.

▸ Histological examination revealed a high-grade transitional cell carcinoma (TCC) that was invading the lamina propria (pathology G3 pT1c).

▸ On re-resection, there was no evidence of any tumour or carcinoma *in situ*. MT was then to be managed with Bacillus Calmette–Guérin (BCG) maintenance, along with regular surveillance cystoscopies. If she were to fail BCG, then she would be managed endoscopically as she is not fit for cystectomy.

▸ She was then discharged and allowed home.

▸ One week ago, MT began to pass large volumes of blood in her urine. She said that she had the desire to urinate, but when she tried she would pass only blood.

▸ After two days, MT began to experience severe suprapubic pain and she was unable to urinate. It is the worst pain that she has ever experienced.

▸ She was subsequently readmitted.

Past medical history

▸ Severe essential tremor (uses a wheelchair/walking frame)

▸ Type 2 diabetes mellitus

▸ Molluscum contagiosum

▸ Keratosis

▸ Gallbladder calculus with acute cholecystitis (gallbladder excised 1985).

Drug history

Drug	Class	Dose	Frequency	Indication
Gliclazide	Sulphonurea	40 mg	od	Type 2 diabetes
Nitrazepam	Benzodiazepine	5 mg	od	Essential tremor
Aspirin	COX inhibitor	75 mg	od	Cardioprotection
Paracetamol	COX inhibitor	1 g	od	Pain
Inderal-LA	Beta-blocker	320 mg	od	Essential tremor

Allergies

▶ NKDA.

Family history

▶ History of essential tremor in her mother and grandmother

▶ No other significant family history.

Social history

▶ MT has been married to her husband for 58 years; they have two daughters (aged 55, 58 years)

▶ She spent her working years in hotel administration and retired 20 years ago; she has never worked with any chemicals

▶ She has smoked 20 cigarettes/day (62 pack-years), and has recently cut down to 10/day

▶ She drinks alcohol occasionally.

Systemic enquiry

▶ **Neurological:** No headaches, faints or fits. No LOC. No weakness or paraesthesia.

▶ **Cardiovascular:** No SOB; no chest pains; no ankle swelling.

▶ **Respiratory:** No cough or haemoptysis.

▶ **Genitourinary:** Haematuria.

▶ **Gastrointestinal:** No change in bowel habit, melaena or PR bleeding.

▶ **Musculoskeletal:** Nil.

Physical examination

General

▸ Rather pale lady, sitting comfortably in her chair

▸ An intention tremor was noted when she reached out to try to touch or use objects

▸ A catheter was in place, and the contents of the bag were rose-coloured

Vital signs

▸ HR 55 bpm – regular

▸ BP 122/75 mmHg

▸ RR 16 breaths/minute

▸ O_2 sats 98%.

Cardiovascular

▸ No visible JVP

▸ Apex beat in fifth intercostal space in the mid-clavicular line

▸ S1, S2; regular rate

▸ Peripheral pulses present

▸ No oedema.

Gastrointestinal/abdominal

▸ Scar in right upper quadrant from previous cholecystectomy

▸ Palpable bladder to the umbilicus

▸ Resonant, tense

▸ No hepatosplenomegaly

▸ Bowel sounds present.

☰ Summary of patient's problems

▸ Haematuria

▸ Severe suprapubic pain.

❓ Questions

▸ Based on the patient's symptoms, what are the main differential diagnoses?

▸ What initial investigations would help confirm the diagnosis?

▸ What is your immediate management plan?

Differential diagnosis

▸ Clot retention

▸ UTI.

Results of investigations

Blood results

▸ Hb 79 g/L (reference range 115–165 g/L)

Renal ultrasound

▸ Both kidneys normal

▸ No evidence of hydronephrosis

▸ Few small cysts in right kidney.

Diagnosis

▸ Clot retention post re-section of bladder tumour.

MT is an 84-year-old smoker with a history of painless macroscopic haematuria. This is bladder cancer until proven otherwise. TURBT revealed a high-grade TCC. 10 days post-resection, she was admitted with haematuria, severe suprapubic pain and acute retention of urine. Her symptoms were due to clot retention.

Management plan

▸ Assess ABCDE

▸ Establish large-calibre IV access

▸ Give 1000 mL of crystalloid if hypotensive

▸ Analgesia

▸ Irrigation catheter to relieve acute symptoms of clot retention

▸ Promote an active diuresis to prevent further clot formation and retention

▸ Blood transfusion (Hb <80 g/L)

▸ Monitor renal function

▸ Monitor fluid balance.

Background information: haematuria

Haematuria may be microscopic or macroscopic. The causes include:

▸ UTI – most common cause, usually associated with lower urinary tract symptoms, especially cystitis

▸ renal stones – often associated with renal colic

▸ malignancy – most likely to be macroscopic; examples include TCC, renal adenocarcinoma and prostate adenocarcinoma

▸ post-interventional – e.g. post-TURP (transurethral resection of the prostate), post-cystoscopy

▸ renal disease, e.g. glomerulonephritis.

If the patient presents with suprapubic colicky pain or acute retention of urine then clots in the bladder or urethra are the likely cause.

Management

Acute management

Establish IV access and give 1000 mL of crystalloid if the patient is hypotensive or tachycardic. An irrigation catheter may be used to relieve clot colic. Send blood samples for testing and transfuse if Hb is <8 g/dL (80 g/L). Commence antibiotics if there is suspicion of infection.

Investigations

▸ Full clinical exam (include PR for prostate)

▸ Kidney ultrasound

▸ Cystoscopy

▸ CT abdomen if a renal tumour is suspected.

Background information: acute urinary retention

Acute urinary retention is the inability to pass urine and is usually associated with pain. The causes, clinical features, investigations and management of acute urinary retention are shown in the table below.

Causes	Clinical features	Investigations	Management
Prostatic enlargement	Suprapubic pain	Urine (M, C & S)	Analgesia
Post-urological surgery	Inability to pass urine	Bloods (FBC, U+Es, creatinine)	Insert catheter
Bladder or stone impaction	May dribble urine in small volumes	Cystoscopy	Treat cause
UTI	Palpable bladder		
Pharmacological (anticholinergics, alpha sympathomimetics, alcohol)	Prostatic enlargement on PR exam		
Loss of neurological control (trauma, epidural, etc.)			

Background information: bladder cancer

The majority of bladder cancers arise from the uroepithelium or transitional cell lining, which it shares in continuum with the renal pelvis and the proximal urethra.

Transitional cell carcinoma

TCC of the bladder is the fifth most common cause of cancer death and the most common form of bladder cancer in the UK. Transitional cell tumours are associated with exposure to aromatic hydrocarbons, which were extensively used in the chemical and dyes industries until their carcinogenic properties were recognised. Thus, workers in the petrochemical, industrial dye and rubber industries and chimney sweeps were historically a high-risk group for the development of bladder cancer. It is also associated with cigarette-smoking, especially in women. It is thought that the risk is due to the excretion of carcinogenic products in the urine. The bladder is more susceptible to urinary carcinogens as urine is stored in the bladder for relatively long periods of time.

TCC is the most common form of bladder cancer. The majority of transition cell tumours are superficial at presentation.

▶ *In situ*: a pre-malignant form associated with increased frequency and dysuria

▶ Superficial 'papilliferous': confined to the mucosa

▶ Invasive: invades through mucosa to bladder wall and potentially further.

Squamous cell carcinoma

Squamous cell carcinoma is usually caused by chronic irritation due to schistosomiasis, indwelling catheter, repeated previous surgical interventions.

Adenocarcinoma

▶ Rare

▶ Presents in middle age

▶ Usually located in the dome of the bladder

▶ Associated with the urachus (runs from the apex of the bladder to the umbilicus, and is usually obliterated at birth).

Clinical features

The majority of cases present with painless haematuria. Bleeding at the end of micturition, and especially the passage of pink/red urine, suggests that the bladder is the site of bleeding. Uniformly dark-coloured urine suggests that the source is the upper tract.

Other features are dysuria, renal colic due to clot retention, disturbance of the urinary stream and retention of urine.

Investigations

▶ Urine cytology – may reveal malignant cells

▶ Cystoscopy

▶ Transurethral resection – the gold standard, permits resection of the tumour and subsequent histological analysis

▶ Upper tract imaging – IVU and renal ultrasound

▶ Magnetic resonance imaging (MRI)/CT – detects local or systemic spread.

Tumour Node Metastases classification of urinary bladder cancer 2017

pT – Primary tumour

pTX Primary tumour cannot be assessed

pT0 No evidence of primary tumour

pTa Non-invasive papillary carcinoma

pTis Carcinoma *in situ*

pT1 Tumour invades subepithelial connective tissue

pT2 Tumour invades muscle

    pT2a Tumour invades superficial muscle (inner half)

    pT2b Tumour invades deep muscle (outer half)

pT3 Tumour invades perivesical tissue

    pT3a Microscopicallly

    pT3b Macroscopicallly (extravesical mass)

pT4 Tumour invades any of the following: prostate, uterus, vagina, pelvic wall or abdominal wall

    pT4a Tumour invades prostate stroma, seminal vesicles, uterus or vagina

    pT4b Tumour invades pelvic wall or abdominal wall

pN – Lymph nodes

pNX Regional lymph nodes cannot be assessed

pN0 No regional lymph node metastasis

pN1 Metastasis in a single lymph node in the true pelvis

pN2 Metastasis in multiple lymph nodes in the true pelvis

pN3 Metastasis in a common iliac lymph node(s)

pM – Distant metastasis

pM1 Distant metastasis

    M1a Non-regional lymph nodes

    M1b Other distant metastasis

The 'P' system (lower-case 'p' for the biopsy specimen and capital 'P' for the whole specimen) classifies the extent of invasion on gross anatomical and histological grounds. The 'G' system grades the lesion according to the degree of differentiation (G1 = well differentiated, G2 = moderately differentiated, G3 = poorly differentiated).

Staging

The TNM clinical system is used in staging bladder tumours.

Treatment

Superficial TCC (Ta, T1)

Small superficial tumours can be treated by endoscopic diathermy alone. However, recurrence is common and regular endoscopic surveillance is recommended. Intravesical chemotherapy with a single dose of mitomycin C instilled after resection of the tumour reduces the risk of tumour recurrence. For multiple or recurrent TCC, six intravesical treatments are given.

Carcinoma *in situ*

This requires thorough therapy to prevent invasive TCC. Immunotherapy with BCG is effective in 60% of cases.

Invasive TCC

Curative therapy can be offered with radical cystectomy (combined with a urinary diversion via an ileal conduit) or radical radiotherapy.

Prognosis

For lesions not involving the bladder muscle, the 5-year survival rate is 80–90%. However, it is thought that approximately 30% will develop invasive disease. The 5-year survival for muscle invasive bladder cancer is 40–50%.

Metastatic disease carries a poor prognosis, with a median survival of only 13 months.

Resources

NICE *Bladder cancer: diagnosis and management, NG2* (2015): www.nice.org.uk/guidance/ng2

Case 17: Bilious vomiting

Presenting complaint

▶ DM is a 46-year-old lady with a past medical history of ovarian carcinoma who presented with vomiting and epigastric discomfort.

History of presenting complaint

▶ DM presented to her GP with a 2-day history of severe RIF pain. Investigations revealed that she had ovarian carcinoma, and she subsequently underwent a laparotomy at which a total abdominal hysterectomy, bilateral salpingo-oophorectomy (BSO) and washings were performed.

▶ It was initially thought that the tumour was a stage 1C ovarian tumour, but pathology, surprisingly, reported that it was of GI origin.

▶ Upper and lower GI endoscopy failed to show any primary site from the GI tract and she was re-referred back to the gynaecological MDT.

▶ She was commenced on a chemotherapy regime that would be active against colorectal and upper GI tumours (ECF – epirubicin, cisplatin and 5-FU [fluorouracil]).

▶ All was thought to be well until 12 weeks ago, when she presented with epigastric discomfort and constant vomiting.

▶ She describes the discomfort as an 'uncomfortable weight' in the epigastric region. It does not radiate and there are no relieving factors. Her appetite has decreased significantly and she has lost 2 stone (12.7 kg) in weight.

▶ She has vomited every day. She has not noticed any haematemesis. Initially she restricted herself to a liquid diet, but this was eventually also intolerable.

▶ She went to her GP who prescribed antiemetics and made a referral to the surgeons.

▶ She was scheduled to be admitted to have an endoscopy, barium meal and follow-through. One week before admission, when she had not opened her bowels for 7 days, she collapsed at home and was brought in as an emergency.

▶ A subsequent laparotomy revealed a lesion at the duodenal–jejunal junction, which looked very typical of a primary carcinoma.

Past medical history

▶ Ovarian cancer– hysterectomy, BSO and washings

▶ Depression

▶ Asthma

▶ No hypertension or diabetes.

Drug history

Drug	Class	Dose	Frequency	Indication
Seretide	Fluticasone propionate	2 puffs	bd	Prophylaxis of asthma
Citalopram	SSRI	60 mg	od	Depression
Salbutamol	Beta-agonist	2 puffs	bd	Prophylaxis of asthma
Lansoprazole	PPI	30 mg	od	GORD Epigastric discomfort
Amitriptyline	Tricyclic antidepressant	10 mg	od	Chemotherapy-related peripheral neuropathy

Allergies

▶ NKDA.

Family history

▶ DM has a positive family history of asthma and type 1 diabetes.

▶ Her father died this year at the age of 68 as a result of thyroid cancer; it has been a particularly difficult time for DM and her family

▶ Her mother is 68 years old and is well

▶ She has three sisters (40, 44, 50) who are also well

▶ She is not aware of any family history of ovarian, breast, endometrial or bowel cancer.

Social history

▶ DM has been married to her husband for 25 years

▶ They have three children (21, 16, 13)

▶ Before becoming unwell, DM worked part-time making blinds; she has not worked for over a year due to her illness

▶ Her husband has arthritis and is also unable to work

▶ She is a non-smoker and does not drink alcohol.

Systemic enquiry

- **Neurological:** No headaches or LOC. Poor vision. Peripheral neuropathy.
- **Cardiovascular:** No chest pain; no breathlessness.
- **Respiratory:** No SOB. No cough or haemoptysis.
- **Genitourinary:** Nil.
- **Gastrointestinal:** GORD; epigastric discomfort; no change in bowel habit.
- **Musculoskeletal:** Nil.

Physical examination

General

- Overweight, middle-aged lady who looks older than her age, sitting comfortably in her chair
- She looks very pale.

Vital signs

- Temp 36.6°C
- HR 80 bpm – regular
- O₂ sats 100% on air.
- BP 130/100 mmHg
- RR 14 breaths/minute

Cardiovascular

- No visible JVP
- S1, S2; regular rate
- No oedema.
- Apex beat in fifth intercostal space in the mid-clavicular line
- Peripheral pulses present

Respiratory

- Chest clear
- No added sounds or wheeze.

Gastrointestinal/abdominal

- No jaundice; very pale.
- There is an old lower abdominal midline scar consistent with previous gynaecological surgery. There is also a new upper abdominal midline scar consistent with a jejunal resection.
- The abdomen is soft and non-tender; no guarding or rebound tenderness.
- Bowel sounds active.

☰ Summary of patient's problems

▸ Epigastric discomfort

▸ Vomiting

▸ Significant weight loss.

❷ Questions

▸ Based on the patient's symptoms, what are the main differential diagnoses?

▸ What initial investigations would help confirm the diagnosis?

▸ What is your immediate management plan?

Differential diagnosis

▶ Small-bowel obstruction (postoperative-related adhesions or malignant due to history of ovarian tumour and surgery)

▶ Gastroenteritis

▶ Inflammatory bowel disease

▶ Pancreatitis

▶ GORD

▶ Large-bowel obstruction

▶ Constipation.

Initial management plan

▶ Assess ABCDE

▶ Establish IV access

▶ Request bloods (FBC, U+Es, LFTs, CRP, amylase)

▶ IV fluids and catheterise

▶ Morphine (5 mg IV) + antiemetic

▶ CXR; abdominal X-ray (AXR) – look for perforation/obstruction

▶ DVT prophylaxis – dalteparin sodium (Fragmin)

▶ NBM + nasogastric (NG) tube

▶ Senior review.

Results of investigations

▶ Bloods showed a mild inflammatory response

▶ AXR showed small-bowel dilatation.

Diagnosis

▶ Small-bowel carcinoma resulting in small-bowel obstruction

DM is a 46-year-old lady who presented with epigastric discomfort and constant bilious vomiting. She had not opened her bowels for 7 days and she collapsed at home. These symptoms are highly suggestive of small-bowel obstruction.

Definitive surgical management

An emergency laparotomy revealed a lesion at the duodenal–jejunal junction that looked very typical of a primary carcinoma. She then had a jejunal resection.

Background information: intestinal obstruction

Any part of the GI tract may become obstructed and present as an acute abdomen. Intestinal obstruction is associated with a high morbidity and mortality if managed incorrectly. It can be broadly classified as shown below, but the main differentiation lies between the small and large bowel.

Classification of intestinal obstruction

Small bowel:

▶ High/low

Large bowel:

▶ Mechanical/functional

▶ Simple/strangulated

▶ Partial/complete

▶ Acute/sub-acute/acute-on-chronic/ chronic.

Mechanical obstruction

A mechanical obstruction results from a physical blockage impeding the passage of bowel contents. These blockages can be divided into extrinsic, intrinsic and those that arise from inside the lumen.

In the UK, the most common cause of small-bowel obstruction is adhesions (60%), followed by hernias (20%) and malignancy (both primary and secondary; 10%).

In the large bowel, malignancy is the most common cause (65%), followed by complicated diverticular disease (10%) and volvulus (5%).

Causes of mechanical obstruction

Intrinsic	Extrinsic	Luminal
Congenital atresia

Inflammatory strictures – Crohn's disease, TB

Tumours – benign, malignant | Adhesions

Hernias

Volvulus

Intussusception

Congenital bands

Inflammatory masses

Tumours | Foreign bodies

Gallstones

Parasites

Bezoars (ball of swallowed foreign material, usually hair or fibre, that collects in the stomach and fails to pass through the intestines) |

Functional obstruction

This form of obstruction results from atony of the intestine with loss of normal peristalsis, in the absence of a mechanical cause. In the small bowel it is usually referred to as paralytic ileus, whereas in the large bowel it is usually referred to as pseudo-obstruction.

Causes of functional obstruction

Metabolic

▶ Hypokalaemia

▶ Hyponatraemia

▶ Hypothermia

▶ Hypoxia

▶ Diabetic ketoacidosis

▶ Uraemia

▶ Dehydration

Drugs

▶ Tricyclic antidepressants

▶ General anaesthesia

Sepsis (acute pancreatitis)
Retroperitoneal malignancy (Ogilvie's syndrome)

Trauma

▶ Head injury

▶ Spinal injury

▶ Pelvic surgery

Local (affecting bowel motility)

▶ Intra-abdominal infection/peritonitis

▶ *Strongyloides* (threadworm)

▶ Postoperative ileus

Clinical features

General

The bowel proximal to the physical obstruction dilates as a result of the accumulation of fluid and gas. Absorption from the lumen is diminished and there is a net loss of water and electrolytes into the bowel lumen, some of which may then be lost in vomiting.

The patient will therefore show signs of dehydration and hypovolaemia, with a decreased skin turgor, dry skin, hypotension and tachycardia. The dilatation of the bowel activates stretch receptors in the wall, resulting in reflex contraction of smooth muscle. This produces colicky abdominal pain and distension.

The bowel distal to the obstruction collapses as gas and fluid no longer pass into it. If the obstruction is not overcome, the reflex activity proximal to the obstruction will eventually cease and the bowel becomes atonic, unless strangulation or perforation occur. In the absence of strangulation or perforation, hypovolaemia and ultimately starvation are the main factors which threaten life.

Increasing small-bowel distension leads to increased intraluminal pressures. This can cause compression of mucosal lymphatics leading to bowel wall lymphoedema. With even higher intraluminal hydrostatic pressures, increased hydrostatic pressure in the capillary beds results in massive third-spacing of fluid, electrolytes and proteins into the intestinal lumen. The fluid loss and dehydration that ensue may be severe and contribute to increased morbidity and mortality.

Vomiting

Colicky pain and vomiting are early features of small-bowel obstruction, with constipation appearing late and distension only really appearing if the obstruction is fairly distal.

The more proximal the obstruction, the earlier the vomiting occurs. It can occur even if nothing is taken by mouth because saliva and other GI secretions continue to be produced and enter the stomach. At least 10 L of fluid are secreted into the GI tract each day.

The nature of the vomit gives important clues to the level of obstruction.

▶ Vomiting of semi-digested food is suggestive of gastric outlet obstruction.

▶ Copious vomiting of bile-stained fluid suggests upper small-bowel obstruction.

▶ Thick and foul-smelling (faeculent) vomitus suggests a more distal obstruction.

Constipation

Distal to the obstruction, bowel gas is absorbed and propulsion of bowel contents is arrested. The resulting absolute constipation or obstipation (neither faeces nor flatus are passed rectally) is pathognomonic of bowel obstruction.

Investigations

▸ Plain abdominal X-ray – small-bowel distension (>2.5 cm in diameter) is suggestive of the diagnosis and resuscitation is instituted

▸ CT will confirm the diagnosis.

Management of intestinal obstruction

▸ Resuscitation – oxygen, venous access, monitor vital signs; oral intake is discontinued and intravenous fluids are given

▸ If the patient is vomiting or there is marked small-bowel dilatation, a NG tube is passed and the gastric contents are aspirated. This will control nausea and vomiting, remove swallowed air and reduce gaseous distension. It will also minimise the risk of inhalation of gastric contents.

▸ Two-thirds of uncomplicated cases are due to adhesions and will usually resolve with conservative measures

▸ Surgery may be required to relieve the obstruction; provided strangulation can be excluded and the caecum is not dangerously distended, surgery can be deferred for 1–2 days

▸ At operation the cause of the obstruction is confirmed and dealt with appropriately.

Resources

Small-bowel obstruction: evaluation and management, J Trauma 2012;73:S362 (doi: 10.1097/ TA.0b013e31827019de)

Case 18: Crohn's disease: abdominal pain and vomiting

Presenting complaint

▶ DP is a 35-year-old male smoker with known Crohn's colitis who presented with a 2-day history of sudden, severe generalised abdominal pain, nausea and vomiting.

History of presenting complaint

▶ DP was recently diagnosed with Crohn's colitis following a barium enema and colonoscopy, although he feels that he has been unwell for many years. He has been managed by his GP since then with mesalazine and steroids.

▶ Two days before admission, he experienced sudden-onset, severe abdominal pain that was aggravated by movement and was partially relieved by lying still in bed.

▶ He had no appetite and felt nauseated. He vomited 7–8 times over 2 days. It was non-projectile and there was no haematemesis. He felt feverish, sweaty and clammy.

▶ He had not opened his bowels in 4 days and he had not passed any flatus. He subsequently phoned NHS 111 and he was admitted to hospital.

Past medical history

▶ *H. pylori*
▶ Asthma (childhood).

Drug history

▶ Mesalazine (Pentasa) – 3 g/day (ongoing)
▶ Prednisolone 40 mg for 2 weeks, then reduced by 5 mg/week.

Family history

▶ His father was diagnosed with colorectal cancer 2 years ago at the age of 58; he is doing well following a resection

▶ Family history of colorectal cancer (DP thinks that his aunt and cousin both had it)

▶ He is an only child; his mother is 62 years old and is well.

Social history

▶ He has recently returned from Amsterdam where he had been living for 2 years, and is currently living with his parents

▶ He smokes 5 cigarettes/day and drinks 30 units/week

▶ He is a freelance computer programmer but has been unable to work recently because of his colitis.

Systemic enquiry

▶ **Neurological:** No headaches, faints, fits or 'funny turns'.

▶ **Cardiovascular:** No chest pain. No SOB.

▶ **Respiratory:** No cough, haemoptysis or sputum production.

▶ **Genitourinary:** Dysuria and frequency.

▶ **Gastrointestinal:** no melaena or fresh PR bleeding. No mucus. No perianal disease.

▶ **Musculoskeletal:** Nil.

Physical examination

General

▶ Alert gentleman who is clearly in pain

▶ He looks thin and pale.

Vital signs

▶ BP 125/80 mmHg

▶ RR 16 breaths/minute

▶ HR 80 bpm – regular

▶ O_2 sats 97% on air

Cardiovascular

▶ No visible JVP

▶ Apex beat in fifth intercostal space in the mid-clavicular line

▶ S1, S2; regular rate

▶ Peripheral pulses present

▶ No oedema

▶ No murmurs.

Respiratory

▶ No use of accessory muscles

▶ Thorax symmetrical; good expansion

▶ Equal air entry

▶ No added sounds.

Gastrointestinal/abdominal

▶ No finger clubbing, Dupuytren's contractures, palmar erythema or koilonychia

▶ No jaundice

▶ No spider naevi

▶ Generally tender, distended abdomen

▶ Bowel sounds active

▶ No guarding or rebound tenderness

▶ No obvious masses or organomegaly

▶ No hernias.

Other

▶ No eye disease (conjunctivitis, iritis, uveitis, episcleritis)

▶ No aphthous ulcers, angular stomatitis or angular chelitis

▶ Tongue normal

▶ Skin: no erythema nodosum or pyoderma gangrenosum; no lymphadenopathy of supraclavicular nodes.

≔ **Summary of patient's problems**

▶ Crohn's disease

▶ Severe abdominal pain

▶ Vomiting

▶ Systemic upset – fever

▶ Constipation and not passing flatus.

---

❷ **Questions**

▶ What are the main differential diagnoses?

▶ What initial investigations would help confirm the diagnosis?

▶ What is your immediate management plan?

Differential diagnosis

- Small-bowel obstruction
- Acute severe colitis
- GORD
- Constipation.
- Perforated bowel
- Pancreatitis
- Large-bowel obstruction

Initial management plan

- Assess ABCDE
- Establish IV access
- Request bloods (FBC, U+Es, LFTs, CRP, amylase)
- IV fluids and catheterise
- Morphine (5 mg IV) + antiemetic
- CXR; AXR – look for perforation/obstruction
- DVT prophylaxis – dalteparin sodium (Fragmin)
- NBM + NG tube
- Senior review.

Results of investigations

Blood results

Substance	Reference range	Result
Na$^+$	135–145 mmol/L	133 mmol/L
K$^+$	3.5–5.0 mmol/L	5.0 mmol/L
Cl$^-$	97–107 mmol/L	99 mmol/L
Urea	2.5–6.7 mmol/L	7.3 mmol/L
Creatinine	40–130 µmol/L	72 µmol/L
Bilirubin	3–17 µmol/L	12 µmol/L
ALT	3–35 U/L	11 U/L
AST	3–35 U/L	19 U/L
Alk phos	40–150 U/L	49 U/L
Hb	115–165 g/L	86 g/L
WCC	4–11 × 10^9/L	15.7 × 10^9/L
CRP	<10 mg/L	105 mg/L

CXR

▶ No free air under the diaphragm.

AXR

▶ Dilated gas-filled loops of small bowel: appearance suggestive of small-bowel obstruction.

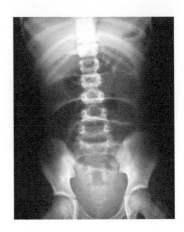

Diagnosis

▶ Small-bowel obstruction secondary to Crohn's disease

DP is a 35-year-old smoker with known Crohn's colitis who presented with a 2-day history of sudden, severe generalised abdominal pain. He felt feverish, sweaty and clammy and he had not opened his bowels or passed any flatus in four days. An AXR suggested small-bowel obstruction.

Definitive surgical management

▶ DP was taken to theatre where he had an extended right hemicolectomy, ileocolic resection and ileostomy.

Background information: Crohn's disease

Inflammatory bowel disease includes Crohn's disease and ulcerative colitis.

Crohn's disease is an idiopathic, chronic, transmural granulomatous inflammatory bowel disease that can affect any part of the GI tract from the mouth to the anus.

Epidemiology

Crohn's disease affects 50–100 people per 100 000. It occurs most often in adults aged 25–40 years, but there is a second peak of incidence after the age of 70. There is a slight female predominance.

Aetiology

The precise aetiology of Crohn's disease is unknown but it has been linked with:

▸ genetics – familial tendency but exact genes are unknown

▸ high-sugar, low-fibre diet

▸ anaerobes

▸ altered cell-mediated immunity.

Cigarette-smoking is the single most important risk factor for developing the disease, and it is also associated with increased disease severity and frequency of relapse, as well as the need for surgical intervention.

Pathology

While the disease can affect any part of the GI tract from the mouth to the anus, it most often affects the terminal ileum (50%) and proximal colon. Normal segments of bowel may be present between grossly diseased areas (skip lesions).

Microscopically, there are deep fissuring ulcers, oedema and inflammatory cell infiltrates with foci of lymphocytes and non-caseating epithelioid granulomas. Although granuloma formation is typical of Crohn's

disease, the diagnosis is not dependent on their presence.

Macroscopically, the disease is characterised by a cobblestone appearance, in which oedematous islands of mucosa are separated by fissures that can extend through all the layers of the bowel wall. Serpiginous ulceration is common. Fibrosis produces strictures of varying number and length. Full-thickness involvement of the wall leads to serosal inflammation, adhesion to neighbouring structures and sinus or fistula formation. Fistulation may be between other loops of bowel, other viscera or the skin. Toxic dilatation can also complicate colonic disease.

Clinical presentation

Crohn's disease is a chronic disorder with exacerbations, remissions and a varied clinical presentation. Patients may present with GI symptoms such as colicky abdominal pain, diarrhoea or perianal disease (e.g. perianal sepsis, abscess or fistulae). One should consider Crohn's disease in all patients with perianal fistulae or sepsis that is resistant to treatment. Patients may also present with symptoms of chronic systemic disease such as weight loss, malnutrition or anaemia. This may present as failure to thrive in children. Furthermore, complications of the disease may be the presenting feature, e.g. acute or chronic intestinal obstruction due to stricturing or fibrostenosing, enteroenteric or enterocutaneous fistulae.

Upon examination, there may be abdominal tenderness and a mass in the RIF. There may also be evidence of perianal disease, such as abscesses or fistulae.

Inflammatory bowel diseases are associated with extraintestinal conditions affecting many systems:

▸ hands – finger clubbing

▸ skin – erythema nodosum, pyoderma gangrenosum, aphthous ulcers of mouth

- eyes – conjunctivitis, iritis, uveitis, episcleritis

- skeletal system – large-joint arthritis, sacroiliitis, ankylosing spondylitis, osteomalacia

- hepatic – fatty liver, gallstones, cholangiocarcinoma

- haematological – megaloblastic or iron-deficiency anaemia, hypercoagulable state.

Differential diagnosis

The disease has many non-specific GI and systemic symptoms, so can be difficult to differentiate from other disorders.

- Ulcerative colitis

- Irritable bowel syndrome (no radiological abnormalities)

- Infective causes of inflammation – *Campylobacter coli, Yersinia enterocolitica, Salmonella typhi*, tuberculous enteritis

- Malabsorption, e.g. coeliac disease

- Diverticular disease

- Small-bowel lymphoma.

In particular, UC too is associated with bloody diarrhoea, but has continuous disease pathology as opposed to Crohn's exacerbating and remitting pattern. Furthermore, UC is more common in non-smokers.

Investigations

- Bloods – FBC (possible iron-deficiency anaemia from chronic blood loss), ESR, CRP (both as monitoring tools rather than diagnostic), U+Es, LFTs, blood culture (exclude infective cause)
Markers of activity – ↓Hb, ↑ESR, ↑CRP, ↑WCC, ↓albumin

- Serology – iron, B12 and red-cell folate (possible anaemia).

- Microbiology – stool samples to exclude infectious causes of diarrhoea

- Barium follow-through (or small-bowel enema) – look for typical appearance of cobblestone mucosa, rose thorn fissures, multiple irregular small-bowel strictures, interloop fistulae and skip lesions

- Flexible sigmoidoscopy or colonoscopy + biopsy to determine the presence and extent of colonic involvement: biopsy of normal rectal tissue may reveal occult large-bowel involvement, especially if there is perianal involvement

- An MRI may be required to assess perianal disease.

Distinctions between Crohn's disease and UC

Feature	Crohn's disease	Ulcerative colitis
Distribution	Commonly terminal ileum May occur anywhere from mouth to anus	Colon, rectum
Skip lesions	Common	Rare
Affected bowel	Thickened wall, narrowed lumen	Mucosal ulceration, dilated lumen
Extent of inflammation	Transmural	Mucosal
Granulomas	Often present	Absent
Fissures and fistulae	Common	Rare
Cancer risk	Slightly increased	Significantly increased

Treatment

The natural history of Crohn's disease, with spontaneous relapses and remissions, makes the evaluation of treatment complicated. Essentially, first-line management is medical, with surgery reserved for those that do not respond to medical therapy or those who develop complications. Steroids and immunosuppressive therapy combined with nutritional support form the cornerstone of medical treatment.

Steroids

▸ Steroids can be used in the acute phase, but every attempt should be made to avoid long-term steroid therapy in view of the risk of complications.

▸ Oral prednisolone for mild attack e.g. 30 mg/day for 1 week then 20 mg/day for 1 month then lower the dose by 5 mg every 2–4 weeks.

▸ IV hydrocortisone, e.g. 100 mg/6 h for severe attack then transfer to oral prednisolone 40 mg if improving after 5 days.

▸ Topical steroids (e.g. hydrocortisone 100 mg in 100 mL 0.9% saline/12 h PR) for rectal disease.

▸ Steroids provide the quickest and most reliable response in active disease.

Aminosalicylates

▸ Slow-release mesalazine releases 5-aminosalicylate proximally in the gut, making it useful in small-bowel disease as well as colitis.

▸ High-dose mesalazine given for 4 months may induce remission in moderately active ileocaecal Crohn's disease.

Immunosuppression

▸ Azathioprine (2–2.5 mg/kg daily) or 6-mercaptopurine (1–1.5 mg/kg daily) can be used in resistant cases to induce remission and also to maintain it (response may take up to 4 months).

▸ Methotrexate (25 mg IM weekly) improves symptoms and reduces steroid requirements in 40% of patients with chronically active steroid-dependent Crohn's disease.

▸ However, there are concerns about complications of long-term immunosuppression and the agents are not generally continued beyond 2 years without review; they are seldom used beyond 4 years.

▸ Monoclonal antibodies to TNF-α (e.g. infliximab) are now frequently used in specialist centres and have a place in patients with fistulating Crohn's disease.

Supportive treatment

▸ Correct anaemia (supplemental iron/ vitamins or transfusion)

▸ Manage malnourishment with high-protein, low-residue or elemental diet

▸ Hydrophilic colloid preparations and codeine phosphate for diarrhoea

▸ Colestyramine to bind bile salts (to prevent their cathartic effects on colon)

▸ Bisphosphonates and vitamin D for osteoporosis

▸ Metronidazole 400 mg/8 h PO or 500 mg/8 h IV (or co-amoxiclav) in perianal disease or superadded infection.

Surgery

Almost all patients with Crohn's disease require surgery at some stage. Surgery may have a role in the acute or chronic management. Indications for surgery include:

▸ failure to respond to drugs (most common)

▸ intestinal obstruction from strictures (as in this patient)

▸ intestinal perforation

▸ local complications (fistulae, abscesses).

Surgery aims to defunction (rest) distal disease, e.g. with temporary ileostomy, or resect limited areas. It is not curative. Uninvolved bowel should be preserved and the residual small-bowel length documented. Stricturoplasty is a useful technique that involves longitudinal division of the strictured small bowel, with closure of the defect transversely to widen the intestinal lumen. Radical surgery is contraindicated, as the risk of recurrence is determined by the natural history of the disease rather than the extent of surgery. The recurrence rate following small-bowel resection is 30%, as opposed to <20% in colonic disease. In perianal Crohn's disease, loculated pus can be drained and radical surgery should be avoided, as the disease tends to recur. Fistulae should be laid open and complex reconstructions avoided.

Short gut syndrome is a complication of multiple or extensive small-bowel surgery. Diarrhoea and malabsorption (particularly of fats) lead to a number of metabolic deficiencies including deficiency in the fat-soluble vitamins (A, D, E and K) and vitamin B12, as well as hyperoxaluria (causing renal calculi) and bile salt depletion (causing gallstones).

Resources

NICE *Crohn's disease: management, NG129* (2019): www.nice.org.uk/guidance/ng129

Chapter 3:

Obstetrics, gynaecology and paediatrics

Case 19:
Abdominal swelling and weight loss

👤 Presenting complaint

▶ MC is a female 67-year-old ex-smoker who presented with a 6-week history of abdominal pain, distension, and vomiting and weight loss.

History of presenting complaint

▶ MC describes the abdominal pain as constant and severe. The pain is localised in the lower abdomen and does not radiate. It is aggravated by eating and she has been avoiding food as a result. The pain is also interfering with MC's sleep and it has often woken her during the night.

▶ Her appetite is very poor and she feels that she has lost 8–9 lbs (3–4 kg) over the past couple of months.

▶ When she manages to eat, she is vomiting. She denies haematemesis.

▶ She describes a 'pressure' in her abdomen which makes her feel like she needs to pass a bowel motion. However, her bowel habit has changed recently with fluctuations between constipation and diarrhoea. There is no melaena. She does report passing bright red blood from her anus at times, which she attributes to haemorrhoids and a fissure.

▶ MC has also noticed that her abdomen has become progressively more distended over the past 3 weeks.

▶ She has a 3-week history of dyspnoea, orthopnoea and occasional episodes of PND. There is no cough, haemoptysis or chest pain.

▶ MC went to her GP and she subsequently underwent endoscopy which revealed a mild chronic gastritis.

▶ However, her symptoms persisted and blood tests revealed an elevated cancer antigen (CA)-125 of 479.

Menstrual history

▶ MC experienced the menopause at the age of 40. However, after 2 years she experienced post-menopausal bleeding and this persisted for 6 years until she was 47 years old.

Past gynaecological history

▶ Dilatation and curettage (D&C)

▶ Nil else.

Past obstetrics history

▶ Two pregnancies which went to term. She had a son and a daughter; both were natural births.

Past medical history

- ▸ Gastritis
- ▸ Type 2 DM
- ▸ Hyperthyroid
- ▸ Asthma.

Drug history

Drug	Class	Dose	Frequency	Indication
Serevent	Long-acting beta-2 agonist	1 puff	bd	Asthma
Ventolin	Short-acting beta-2 agonist	2 puffs	bd	Asthma
Beclometasone	Corticosteroid	2 puffs	bd	Asthma
Metformin	Biguanide	500 mg	od	Type 2 DM
Thyroxine	Hormone	50 mg	od	Hyperthyroid
Bendroflumethiazide	Loop diuretic	5 mg	od	Ascites
Simvastatin	Statin	40 mg	nocte	Hyperlipidaemia

Allergies

- ▸ NKDA.

Family history

- ▸ MC has a strong family history of cancer
- ▸ Her father died when he was 59, due to lung cancer
- ▸ Her mother is 97 and still well; MC said that her mother had a 'mass' removed from the skin on her leg some years ago
- ▸ She had a brother who passed away at the age of 40 from prostate cancer and a sister who died at the age of 67 from lung cancer
- ▸ There is no known history of bowel cancer, endometrial, breast or ovarian cancer.

Social history

- ▸ MC was previously married but was divorced over 30 years ago
- ▸ MC has a son who is 45 years old, and two grandchildren who live with her son's ex-wife
- ▸ Her daughter passed away 8 years ago when she was only 35 years old: she had UC and had gone into hospital for a stoma reversal, but two days after the procedure she developed sepsis and unfortunately died

▸ MC lives in a three-bedroom house with her 18-year-old granddaughter, who has 'learning difficulties'; MC is the main carer for her granddaughter since her daughter died, and she is extremely concerned about the granddaughter's care since her diagnosis

▸ She is an ex-smoker, having stopped 7 years ago; she previously smoked 20/day for 40 years (40 pack-years)

▸ She is a non-drinker.

Systemic enquiry

▸ **Neurological:** No falls, LOC, seizures or dizziness. Occasional headaches.

▸ **Cardiovascular:** No ankle oedema or chest pain.

▸ **Respiratory:** Dyspnoea, orthopnoea, PND.

▸ **Genitourinary:** Nil.

▸ **Gastrointestinal:** Change in bowel habit (fluctuates between constipation and diarrhoea). No melaena. Generalised abdominal pain. Nausea and vomiting. Poor appetite.

▸ **Musculoskeletal:** Nil.

Physical examination

General

▸ MC looks tired, extremely pale, unwell and rather cachexic.

Vital signs

▸ Temp 37°C
▸ HR 100 bpm, regular
▸ BP 139/81 mmHg
▸ RR 18 breaths/minute.

Neurological

▸ Patient is orientated to person, time and place

▸ Motor: Good bulk and tone; strength is 5/5 throughout

▸ Cerebellar: finger–nose, heel–shin and rapid alternating movement responses are intact.

Cardiovascular

▸ No visible JVP
▸ No murmurs
▸ Unable to palpate apex beat
▸ No ankle oedema
▸ S1, S2; regular rate
▸ Feels cold and looks very pale.

Respiratory

▸ No use of accessory muscles
▸ Vesicular breath sounds
▸ Tachypnoea
▸ Dyspnoeic at rest.

Gastrointestinal/abdominal

▸ Gross abdominal distension with a drain *in situ* in the left side of the abdomen

▸ No scarring of the abdomen

▸ No jaundice or hepatic flap

▸ The abdomen was soft, with tenderness around the drain area and under the right costal margin

▸ Unable to palpate the liver edge due to pain

▸ Bowel sounds present

▸ No lymphadenopathy.

Musculoskeletal

▸ Full range of movement in all joints; no deformities.

Other

▸ A pelvic, rectal and breast exam should also be carried out.

☰ Summary of patient's problems

▸ Abdominal pain and distension

▸ Weight loss

▸ Raised CA-125.

❓ Questions

▸ What are the main differential diagnoses?

▸ What initial investigations would help confirm the diagnosis?

▸ What is your immediate management plan?

Differential diagnosis

▶ Ovarian cancer

▶ Other cancers, including cancer of the cervix, uterus, rectum and bladder

▶ Other causes of abdominal distension or bloating, such as:

> uterine fibroids, ascites secondary to cirrhosis of the liver, or heart failure

> adenomyosis (gynaecological condition characterised by the abnormal presence of endometrial tissue within the myometrium)

▶ Other causes of early satiety, such as gastric cancer

▶ Other causes of urinary frequency or urgency, such as recurrent UTIs.

▶ Other causes of altered bowel habit, such as:

> irritable bowel syndrome

> constipation (functional or drug-induced)

> coeliac disease

> inflammatory bowel disease

> GI infection

▶ Other causes of abdominal pain or discomfort, such as:

> adhesions

> pelvic inflammatory disease (PID)

> diverticular disease

> chronic pancreatitis

> gallstones

▶ Other causes of a raised serum CA-125, including:

> peritoneal trauma, disease or irritation

> other cancers, such as primary peritoneal cancer, lung cancer and pancreatic cancer

> endometriosis

> PID

> ovarian cyst torsion, rupture or haemorrhage

> pregnancy

> heart failure.

Investigations

▶ Bloods (FBC, U+Es, LFTs, TFTs, CRP, CA-125)

▶ CT abdo/pelvis.

Results of investigations

Blood results

Substance	Reference range	Result
Na$^+$	135–145 mmol/L	136 mmol/L
K$^+$	3.5–5.0 mmol/L	4.4 mmol/L
Cl$^-$	96–105 mmol/L	95 mmol/L
HCO$_3^-$	24–29 mmol/L	26 mmol/L
Urea	2.5–7.8 mmol/L	7.8 mmol/L
Creatinine	55–120 µmol/L	78 µmol/L
Glucose	4.0–7.0 mmol/L	9 mmol/L
AST	<37 U/L	20 U/L
ALT	<40 U/L	13 U/L
Alk phos	30–130 U/L	62 U/L
Bilirubin	F <17 µmol/L, M <21 µmol/L	10 µmol/L
Amylase	<100 U/L	42 U/L
CRP	<10 mg/L	150 mg/L
CA-125	<30 U/mL	479 U/mL
Carcinoembryonic antigen		<1 mcg/L
Hb	135–155 g/L	141 g/L

CT

- Malignant ascites
- Pelvic peritoneal nodules
- Small left pleural effusion
- Small solid area in the left adnexa.

Diagnosis

- Ovarian cancer

MC is a 67-year-old ex-smoker with a strong family history of cancer who presented with a 6-week history of constant lower abdominal pain, vomiting, change in bowel habit and weight loss. Examination revealed gross ascites and generalised abdominal tenderness. Investigations revealed an elevated CA-125 and a CT of the abdomen/pelvis showed a small solid area in the left adnexa indicating ovarian carcinoma.

Management plan

▶ Always assess ABCDE

▶ Analgesia

▶ Antiemetic

▶ IV fluids

▶ Discuss with patient the impact of the diagnosis and offer support

▶ Stage cancer

▶ Gynaecological oncology referral

▶ Discuss at MDT.

Ethical issues and communication skills

MC was transferred to the gynaecological unit unaware of her diagnosis despite the diagnosis being made prior to the referral. This raises a multitude of ethical and moral issues.

▶ **Respect for autonomy:** This includes involving competent patients in healthcare decisions; informing them so they can make decisions; and respecting their views.

▶ **Beneficence (and non-maleficence):** MC's consultant should do what is best for her (and not inflict harm).

▶ **Doctor/patient relationship:** Patients should be informed and fully involved in the management decisions of their care.

▶ **Doctor's duty of care.**

The GMC states that 'relationships based on openness, trust and good communication will enable you to work in partnership with your patients to address their individual needs'. The patient's autonomy was not respected in this case as she was not initially informed about the true gravity of her condition.

Background information: ovarian cancer

Epidemiology

In the Western world, ovarian cancer is the fourth most common cause of death from malignant disease in women after lung, bowel and breast cancer. In the UK it represents 4% of all newly diagnosed cancers, which equates to around 7500 new cases per year. Ovarian tumours are either epithelial or non-epithelial; epithelial tumours account for approximately 90% of tumours.

The incidence of the disease increases with age and is rare under the age of 30 (5/100 000 population). The incidence in women over 45 is approximately 40/100 000.

Epithelial ovarian cancer is often described as a 'silent killer' as in over 60% of cases advanced disease is found at the first presentation. Survival is dependent on the stage of the cancer at initial presentation. Stage 1 disease has a 5-year survival of 85%, whilst stage 4 cancer has a 5-year survival of only about 10%. In the UK the overall 5-year survival is approximately 40%, and over 3000 women die from the disease each year.

Aetiology

The aetiology is unknown, but a number of risk factors have been identified. These include:

▶ nulliparity

▶ positive family history of breast and ovarian cancer (although >90% are spontaneous)

▶ the number of ovulatory cycles experienced in a lifetime – increases with early menarche, late menopause, first child after the age of 30.

Use of the combined oral contraceptive pill and breastfeeding are protective factors.

Pathology of ovarian tumours

The pathology of ovarian tumours can be subdivided into:

▶ epithelial (>90% of ovarian tumours)

▶ germ cell

▶ sex cord/stromal

▶ miscellaneous and metastatic.

Epithelial tumours can be further subdivided:

▶ serous (50%)

▶ endometrioid (30%)

▶ mucinous (20%).

The natural history of the disease is not well understood. Some tumours grow to large cystic structures while others metastasise widely throughout the peritoneum. The tumours can often produce large amounts of ascitic fluid, which can accumulate in the peritoneal cavity and lead to abdominal distension.

Symptoms

Ovarian cancer usually presents by virtue of an expanding intra-abdominal mass causing pain and distension. In the early stages of the disease, it may present with vague symptoms which are often ignored by the patient, and if they are reported to the GP, they are often dismissed. Think of ovarian cancer if these symptoms are present:

▶ abdominal bloating

▶ increased abdominal girth

▶ indigestion, lack of appetite

▶ change in bowel habits

▶ constipation

▶ urinary frequency or incontinence

▶ fatigue

▶ abdominal pain and/or pelvic pain.

92% of women with invasive ovarian tumours and 84% of borderline cases have symptoms with a median duration of 4 months. While reported symptoms can be extremely difficult to differentiate from other, benign conditions, in proven cases of ovarian cancer bloating, fullness and pressure in the abdomen are much more likely to be constant rather than intermittent. In this case, MC's chief complaint was a constant feeling of pressure in her abdomen. Symptoms lasting more than one month should be investigated, and a high level of suspicion is a useful adjunct in making the diagnosis of ovarian cancer, particularly:

▶ in women with a family history of ovarian cancer

▶ in women over 45 years of age

▶ where symptoms appear to persist in the absence of any alternative explanation.

Investigations and diagnosis

If ovarian cancer is suspected, the patient should be referred for an urgent gynaecological opinion. The investigations of choice are ultrasound (most often CT) and CA-125.

Staging

Staging of ovarian cancer is important in determining both prognosis and the method of management. It is based on the FIGO (International Federation of Gynecology and Obstetrics) classification system and is outlined in the table below.

FIGO classification of ovarian carcinoma

Stage I	Growth limited to ovaries only
Stage IA	One ovary, no ascites, no tumour on external surface, capsule intact
Stage IB	Both ovaries involved, no ascites, no tumour on external surface, capsule intact
Stage IC	IA or IB with tumour on surface, capsule ruptured, malignant ascites or positive washings
Stage II	Pelvic extension only
Stage IIA	Extension and/or metastasis to uterus and/or fallopian tubes
Stage IIB	Extension to other pelvic tissues
Stage IIC	IIA or IIB with tumour on surface or capsule ruptured, malignant ascites or positive washings
Stage III	Tumour involving one or both ovaries with peritoneal implants outside the pelvis and/or positive retroperitoneal or inguinal nodes
Stage IIIA	Tumour grossly limited to the true pelvis with negative nodes but histologically confirmed microscopic seeding of abdominal peritoneal surfaces
Stage IIIB	Tumour involving one or both ovaries, histologically confirmed implants on abdominal peritoneal surfaces <2 cm
Stage IIIC	Abdominal implants >2 cm and/or positive retroperitoneal or inguinal nodes
Stage IV	Growth involving one or both ovaries with distant metastasis. If pleural effusion present, positive cytology; parenchymal liver metastasis

Prognosis

Stage	5-year survival
IA, IB, IC	85% overall, 95% for stage IA
IIA, IIB, IIC	30–57%
IIIA, IIIB, IIIC	10–28%
IV	<10%

Management

Treatment is based on surgical excision or debulking (cytoreductive surgery) and chemotherapy.

Resources

NICE *Ovarian cancer: recognition and initial management, CG122* (2011): www.nice.org.uk/guidance/cg122

Case 20: Placenta praevia

Presenting complaint

▶ JM is a 40-year-old para 2+1 who presented at 34 weeks gestation. Her estimated date of delivery (EDD) is 6th May.

History of presenting complaint

Current pregnancy

▶ Her pregnancy has been unremarkable to date and she feels that her baby is very active with good foetal movements. She has no health complaints.

▶ However, at the 20-week scan the placenta was noted to be low-lying. She was re-scanned at 34 weeks. This scan showed grade IV placenta praevia and she was admitted to the antenatal ward as a precaution as she lives more than 3 hours away from the nearest hospital.

▶ She did not experience any pain or discharge.

▶ She experienced a small-volume PV bleed.

Past obstetric history

▶ JM has two children. Her son is 11 years old and her daughter is 7 years old.

▶ JM had a miscarriage 12 months ago when she was 8 weeks pregnant.

Child	Birth weight	Gestation	Type of birth	Duration of labour	Breastfed?
Son	7 lb 8 oz (3.40 kg)	38+1 weeks	Ventouse – baby distressed	12 hours	No
Daughter	6 lb 9 oz (2.98 kg)	39+2 weeks	normal	5–6 hours (induced)	No

Past gynaecological history

▶ JM and her partner were trying for a baby for 5 months before they conceived. Previous to this she was taking the contraceptive pill (Cerazette 75 mg od).

▶ She has regular smears. Her last smear was last year, and she got the result the same day that she found out she was pregnant. The smear showed mild dyskaryosis and unfortunately 7 weeks later JM miscarried. This was a difficult time for JM. Subsequent colposcopy was indicative of 'infection'. She then became pregnant again and so has been asked to return to the clinic for review 6 weeks post-partum.

Past medical history

▶ Asthma

▶ Temporal lobe epilepsy – before conceiving, JM was taking Epilim (500 mg od); her last seizure was 4 years ago

▶ Migraine

▶ IBS

▶ No history of diabetes, hypertension or thyroid disease.

Drug history

Drug	Class	Dose	Frequency	Indication
Seretide	Corticosteroid	1 puff	bd	Asthma
Ventolin	Short-acting beta-2 agonist	2 puffs	bd	Asthma

Allergies

▶ NKDA.

Family history

▶ No significant family history.

Social history

▶ JM is divorced and has been in a relationship with her current partner for 18 months

▶ They had been trying to conceive for 5 months before they were successful

▶ She previously worked as a bookkeeper, but is not working at present

▶ She has never smoked and is a 'social' drinker, but has not drunk alcohol since becoming pregnant.

Systemic enquiry

▶ **Neurological:** No falls, LOC, seizures or dizziness.

▶ **Cardiovascular:** minimal ankle oedema.

▶ **Respiratory:** No dyspnoea, orthopnoea or PND. No cough.

▶ **Genitourinary:** Nil.

▶ **Gastrointestinal:** No change in bowel habit.

▶ **Musculoskeletal:** Nil.

Physical examination

General

▸ JM is sitting comfortably in bed and appears well.

Vital signs

▸ Temp 37°C
▸ BP 127/81 mmHg

▸ HR 80 bpm, regular
▸ RR 16 breaths/minute.

Cardiovascular

▸ No visible JVP
▸ S1, S2; regular rate; no murmurs

▸ Unable to palpate apex beat
▸ Well perfused.

Respiratory

▸ No use of accessory muscles
▸ Vesicular breath sounds.

Other

Due to placenta praevia, no pelvic exam or palpation of the abdomen to determine fundal height and foetal lie, presentation and position was possible.

☰ Summary of patient's problems

▸ PV bleeding
▸ Placenta praevia.

❓ Questions

▸ What are the main differential diagnoses of PV bleeding in pregnancy?
▸ What investigation would help confirm the diagnosis?
▸ What is your immediate management plan?

Differential diagnosis

PV bleeding in pregnancy – in the first trimester:

▶ miscarriage

> ➤ threatened miscarriage: with or without identifiable subchorionic haemorrhage

> ➤ missed miscarriage

> ➤ incomplete miscarriage

▶ subchorionic haemorrhage

▶ ectopic pregnancy

▶ gestational trophoblastic disease

▶ demise of a twin

▶ implantation bleeding.

In the second and third trimesters:

▶ placental abruption

▶ placenta praevia

▶ gestational trophoblastic disease

▶ vasa praevia

▶ uterine rupture.

Results of investigations

▶ Ultrasound – indicative of grade IV placenta praevia.

Diagnosis

▶ Placenta praevia

JM is a 40-year-old para 2+1 who presented at 34 weeks gestation after her 20-week scan was indicative of a low-lying placenta. A repeat scan at 34 weeks showed grade IV placenta praevia.

Management plan

▶ Admit to the ward

▶ FBC

▶ Group and save serum

▶ Discuss significance of placenta praevia and other associated risks with the patient.

Background information: antepartum haemorrhage

Antepartum haemorrhage is bleeding from the genital tract in pregnancy after the 24th week of pregnancy and before the onset of labour.

Causes

▸ Unexplained (97%) – usually marginal placental bleeds (i.e. minor placental abruptions)

▸ Placenta praevia (1%)

▸ Placental abruption (1%)

▸ Other causes (1%) include:

> maternal – incidental (cervical/ectropion)

> maternal – local infection of cervix/vagina

> maternal – genital tract tumours

> maternal – varicosities

> maternal – trauma

> foetal – vasa praevia.

Background information: placenta praevia

The placenta is said to be praevia when all or part of the placenta implants in the lower uterine segment and therefore lies in front of or near the cervical opening. Placenta praevia occurs in 1% of all pregnancies.

Grading

Grading of placenta praevia is important as major degrees of placenta praevia are likely to require operative delivery whereas minor degrees may not prevent successful vaginal delivery. It is also important in making management decisions, because the incidence of morbidity and mortality in the foetus and mother increases as the grade increases. Classically, placenta praevia is divided into four types or grades. Types I and II are regarded as minor and types III and IV as major degrees of placenta praevia.

Gradings for placenta praevia

Type I	The placenta encroaches into the lower uterine segment and lies within 5 cm of the internal cervical os
Type II	The placenta reaches the cervical os but does not cover it
Type III	The placenta covers the cervical os but the placental site is asymmetric, with most of the placenta being on one side of the cervical os
Type IV	The placenta is centrally located over the cervical os

Aetiology and associated factors

Placenta praevia is caused by implantation of the blastocyst low in the uterine cavity. Factors associated with the development of placenta praevia include:

▸ increasing maternal parity

▸ increasing maternal age

▸ increasing placental size (i.e. multiple pregnancy)

▸ endometrial damage (previous D&C)

▸ previous caesarean section

▸ uterine scars and pathology (previous myomectomy and endometritis)

▸ previous placenta praevia

▸ smoking.

Clinical presentation and diagnosis

The main symptom is painless vaginal bleeding. In cases associated with placental abruption there may also be some mild lower abdominal pain. The signs of placenta praevia are:

▸ vaginal bleeding – women classically present with minor degrees of painless vaginal bleeding in the absence of labour pains

- malpresentation of the foetus – the presence of the placenta in the lower segment pushes the presenting part upwards, causing it to lie obliquely or transversely

- uterine hypotonus.

Most women in the UK have a routine scan at 21–23 weeks. In some, the placenta will be low-lying and so they will require a repeat scan later in pregnancy, typically at 34–36 weeks. The diagnosis of placenta praevia is most commonly made on ultrasound.

Management

If the pregnancy is less than 37 weeks then the aim is to treat conservatively. Conservative management of placenta praevia involves admitting the mother to hospital with blood cross-matched until foetal maturity is adequate, and then delivering the child by caesarean section.

Conservative management should be followed unless the bleeding becomes more severe or persistent. The condition can be very serious and bleeding is unpredictable.

If the delivery seems as though it is going to be preterm, then steroids may be given to accelerate maturation of the foetal lungs.

If the pregnancy proceeds to 37–38 weeks then the degree of placenta praevia can be confirmed by vaginal examination. Vaginal examination should be performed only in theatre prepared for caesarean section, with blood cross-matched. Four units of cross-matched blood should be kept ready, even if the mother has never experienced vaginal bleeding.

Resources

RCOG *Placenta praevia and placenta accreta: diagnosis and management, GTG27a* (2018): www.rcog.org.uk/en/guidelines-research-services/guidelines/gtg27a

Case 21: PV bleeding in early pregnancy

👤 Presenting complaint

▶ SR is a 34-year-old lady at 13 weeks gestation who presents with a 2-day history of brown vaginal discharge, PV bleeding and lower abdominal pain.

History of presenting complaint

▶ SR noticed she had been having some brown discharge and she was seen by her GP.

▶ Her GP organised an ultrasound for the next day. However, that night she experienced lower abdominal pain which radiated to her left lower back. The pain was like a cramp and it was partially relieved by co-codamol.

▶ This prompted SR to self-present to the early pregnancy assessment service, but she was told to return the next day as the scan was arranged for then.

▶ At 00:30 that night, she had a gush of fresh PV blood and more lower abdominal cramping, and was brought to hospital via ambulance.

Menstrual history

▶ Menarche – 12/13 years old.

▶ Last menstrual period (LMP) 15 weeks ago

▶ She describes them as heavy for the first 2–3 days and then they gradually become lighter

▶ She has had episodes of flooding in the past

▶ Mild pain in the first 2 days of menstruation, relieved by paracetamol.

Past obstetrics history

Child	Birth weight	Gestation	Type of birth	Duration of labour	Breastfed?
Girl	>7 lb (3.17 kg)	39+2 weeks	Normal vaginal	4–5 hours	No
Girl	>7 lb (3.17 kg)	40 weeks	Normal vaginal	2–3 hours	No

▶ SR had no prenatal complications prior to the birth of her daughters. She had a vaginal tear after the birth of her first child.

▶ She had a miscarriage 11 years ago when she was 8 weeks pregnant. She had another miscarriage last September at 12 weeks gestation.

Past gynaecological history

▶ Previously used the combined oral contraceptive pill for 2–3 years.

Past medical history

▸ Nil.

Drug history

Drug	Class	Dose	Frequency	Indication
Co-codamol	Paracetamol + codeine phosphate	30/500 mg	qds	Pain
Ferrous sulphate	Iron supplement	200 mg	od	Anaemia

Allergies

▸ NKDA.

Family history

▸ No significant family history.

Social history

▸ SR lives with her husband and her two daughters (13 and 11 years old) in a two-bedroom flat.

▸ She is a part-time shop-keeper.

▸ She and her husband have been trying for a baby since last June. She unfortunately miscarried in September. She fell pregnant again in January.

▸ She is a traditional Muslim and is very keen to have a boy. She says that she will keep trying to conceive until she has a boy.

Systemic enquiry

▸ **Neurological:** Nil.   ▸ **Genitourinary:** Nil.

▸ **Cardiovascular:** Nil.   ▸ **Gastrointestinal:** Nil.

▸ **Respiratory:** Nil.   ▸ **Musculoskeletal:** Nil.

Physical examination

General

▸ SR is sitting comfortably in bed.

Vital signs

▸ BP 132/84 mmHg   ▸ RR 14 breaths/minute.

▸ HR 80 bpm, regular

Gastrointestinal/abdominal

▸ Soft and non-tender   ▸ Bowel sounds active.

▸ No organomegaly

Pelvic

▸ Speculum – fresh PV blood   ▸ Multiple small clots removed.

▸ Cervix not visualised

☰ Summary of patient's problems

▸ Early pregnancy

▸ Brown vaginal discharge, PV bleeding and lower abdominal pain.

❓ Questions

▸ What are the main differential diagnoses?

▸ What initial investigations would help confirm the diagnosis?

▸ What is your immediate management plan?

Differential diagnosis

Bleeding in the first trimester:

▶ miscarriage

> ❯ threatened miscarriage with or without identifiable subchorionic haemorrhage

> ❯ missed miscarriage

> ❯ incomplete miscarriage

▶ subchorionic haemorrhage   ▶ demise of a twin

▶ ectopic pregnancy   ▶ implantation bleeding

▶ gestational trophoblastic disease.

Bleeding in second and third trimesters:

▶ placental abruption   ▶ vasa praevia

▶ placenta praevia   ▶ uterine rupture

▶ gestational trophoblastic disease.

Management plan

▶ As always, assess every patient using ABCDE

▶ IV access and bloods, including β-human chorionic gonadotrophin (β-hCG)

▶ Review bloods – check Hb (ensure not anaemic)

▶ Ultrasound.

Diagnosis

▶ Miscarriage

SR is a 34-year-old lady at 13 weeks gestation. She is para 2+2 and presents with a 2-day history of brown discharge, lower abdominal pain and fresh PV bleeding. An ultrasound confirmed that she had miscarried.

Further management plan

The miscarriage was complete, so no specific treatment is needed. Management will involve supportive measures.

Background information: miscarriage

Spontaneous miscarriage is the termination of pregnancy before the 24th week of pregnancy. It is thought to occur in 10–20% of pregnancies and accounts for 50 000 inpatient admissions in the UK each year. There are various clinical types of miscarriage that differ in their presentation.

Types of miscarriage

Threatened miscarriage

The first sign of a threatened miscarriage is the development of vaginal bleeding. This blood loss is not usually accompanied by pain and it occurs before the 24th week. Examination reveals an enlarged uterus and the cervical os is closed. In the past, bed rest was recommended as treatment; however, there is no evidence that it affects the outcome. An ultrasound scan should be carried out to determine whether the pregnancy is still viable, and if it is the mother can be reassured.

Inevitable miscarriage

The patient develops lower abdominal pain, which is usually accompanied by increasing blood loss. Miscarriage is inevitable, because uterine contractions have begun which cause the cervix to dilate. This may be detected on vaginal examination. Surgical evacuation of the uterus is the treatment of choice.

Complete miscarriage

When a miscarriage is complete, the woman experiences uterine contractions, the cervix dilates and blood is lost. The foetus and placenta are expelled together, the uterus contracts and the bleeding subsequently subsides. This type of miscarriage is more common after 16 weeks gestation. As the miscarriage is complete, no further treatment is needed.

Incomplete miscarriage

A miscarriage is said to be incomplete when, in spite of uterine contractions and dilation of the cervix, only the foetus and part of the membranes are expelled. As the placenta remains partially attached to the uterine wall, bleeding may continue for some time. The patient is often in significant pain due to contractions, and there is a lot of blood loss. Examination of the vagina often reveals foetal tissue and blood clots. The bleeding may be managed by administering an intramuscular injection of ergometrine (0.5 mg). Ergometrine decreases blood loss via activation of alpha-adrenoceptors on blood vessels, which leads to vasoconstriction. The pain may be managed with morphine. However, surgical evacuation will ultimately be required and the bleeding may be so severe as to warrant a blood transfusion.

Septic miscarriage

Following miscarriage, the uterus may become infected. Clinically, the findings are similar to those of incomplete miscarriage with the addition of uterine and adnexal tenderness. Signs of shock may also be apparent.

Missed miscarriage

This is the term used to describe the retention of a foetus for a period of several weeks after its death. There may be some vaginal bleeding and the symptoms of pregnancy subside. A negative pregnancy test and ultrasound finding are diagnostic.

If the products are left for an extended period then the gestation may become:

▶ a carneous mole – lobulated mass of laminated blood clot

▶ a macerated foetus – skull bones collapse; spine is flexed; very little amniotic fluid on ultrasound; degeneration of internal organs; abdomen is filled with blood-stained fluid; skin easily peeled.

Most will be expelled spontaneously, but in cases of foetal death of more than four weeks, treatment is as outlined below.

Aetiology

In many cases the cause of the miscarriage remains unknown. Known causes for early pregnancy loss include:

▶ **Genetic abnormalities** – In any form of spontaneous miscarriage up to 55% of products of conception will have an abnormal karyotype. These are usually trisomies (most common), polyploidies or monosomies.

▶ **Maternal condition** – Severe maternal illness associated with infections predisposes to miscarriage. Deficiencies of progesterone and hCG have also been linked to an increased risk of pregnancy loss. Chronic maternal illness involving the cardiovascular, renal and hepatic systems may also result in miscarriage.

▶ **Abnormalities of the uterus** – Congenital abnormalities of the uterus (see figure) may result in miscarriage. Uterine abnormalities are present in 15–30% of women who miscarry. The presence of fibroids may also predispose to early pregnancy loss.

▶ **Cervical incompetence** – This may be congenital but most cases are a result of damage during labour or due to mechanical dilatation. Cervical incompetence means that the uterus is incapable of containing the products of conception and the miscarriage is usually rapid, painless and bloodless.

▶ **Autoimmune factors** – Antiphospholipid antibodies (lupus anticoagulant and anticardiolipin antibodies) are present in 15% of women who miscarry.

Congenital abnormalities of the uterus:

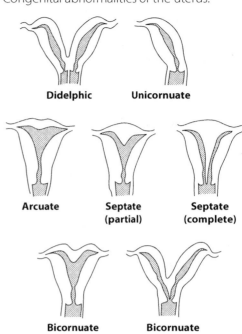

Differential diagnosis

Differential diagnosis of miscarriage is usually straightforward but should include:

▶ ectopic pregnancy

▶ hydatidiform mole

▶ some menstrual disorders.

Management

Transvaginal scanning will be required in the majority of women referred to an early pregnancy assessment service. Ultrasound assessment is particularly reliable in confirming the diagnosis of complete miscarriage (positive predictive value 98%). Urinary hCG is also useful. If the patient is pyrexial, then vaginal swabs should be taken. If the miscarriage is complicated by haemorrhage and infection, then a blood transfusion and broad-spectrum antibiotic therapy may be needed. Pain relief is also required.

Non-sensitised rhesus (Rh) negative women should receive anti-D immunoglobulin in the following situations: ectopic pregnancy, all miscarriages over 12 weeks of gestation (including threatened) and all miscarriages where the uterus is evacuated (whether medically or surgically). Anti-D immunoglobulin should only be given for threatened miscarriage under 12 weeks of gestation when bleeding is heavy or associated with pain. It is not required for cases of complete miscarriage under 12 weeks of gestation when there has been no formal intervention to evacuate the uterus.

Surgical management

Surgical uterine evacuation (evacuation of retained products of conception – ERPC) involves dilatation of the cervix and suction curettage to remove the conceptus. Until recently, up to 88% of women who miscarried were offered ERPC. It remains the treatment of choice if there is excessive and persistent bleeding, if vital signs are unstable or if retained, infected tissue is present.

Medical management

Medical methods are an effective alternative in the management of confirmed first-trimester miscarriage. The natural process of expelling the products of conception from the uterus can be expedited by the use of a prostaglandin analogue such as misoprostol or gemeprost with or without antiprogesterone priming (mifepristone). The products will normally be passed 48–72 hours later. If bleeding persists, an evacuation under general anaesthetic may be needed.

Conservative management

This is the management option of choice for incomplete miscarriages where the uterus is small or when minimal products remain in the uterus.

Resources

NICE *Ectopic pregnancy and miscarriage: diagnosis and initial management, NG 126* (2019): www.nice.org.uk/guidance/ng126

Case 22: Abdominal pain and PV bleeding

👤 Presenting complaint

▶ HM is a 48-year-old lady who presented with a 4-month history of left lower abdominal pain and a 6-week history of haematuria and PV bleeding.

History of presenting complaint

▶ HM went to her GP complaining of severe pain in her left iliac fossa. She was told that she had a 'urine infection or a kidney infection' and was given a course of antibiotics.

▶ The pain persisted and a urine sample confirmed haematuria. Two months later, HM said that she was unable to move due to abdominal pain and she was admitted to hospital. The pain radiated to her left lower back and she describes it as 'severe', grading it as 8/10. It was constant and she felt that it was 'worse than labour'. It often woke her from her sleep and it was accompanied by nausea. Her sleep was grossly disturbed and she had no appetite. She was unsure if she had lost any weight. She had various urological investigations and was sent home.

▶ Two days later, whilst at home with her 12-year-old daughter, HM experienced heavy PV bleeding. She says the bleeding was very heavy and it pooled on the floor. This understandably caused HM and her daughter a great deal of distress. She was then readmitted to hospital.

Menstrual history

▶ Menarche – 12 years

▶ LMP – unsure due to irregular PV bleeding

▶ Periods are initially heavy then light

▶ No period pain

▶ Three episodes of flooding; given maternity pads when admitted

▶ First episode of intermenstrual bleeding 6 weeks ago

▶ Clots.

Past obstetrics history

▶ HM is para 7+1. She has five daughters and two sons. She had a stillbirth at 24 weeks with her first pregnancy when she was 19 years old. She attributed this to 'premature labour'.

▶ Five of her children were home births. She said that they were booked in for hospital deliveries but the labour was so short that it happened at home. She says that all of her labours were less than 30 minutes. All her children weighed over 8 lb (3.63 kg).

▶ She was sterilised after the birth of her last child.

Past gynaecological history

▸ HM's only previous gynaecology intervention was for a laparoscopic sterilisation after the birth of her youngest daughter.

▸ Last smear was 13 years ago.

▸ She said that she was never called for a smear. Despite all her previous admissions, she never had a speculum exam or was offered a smear.

▸ She occasionally used condoms as contraception.

Past medical history

▸ Respiratory symptoms including SOB and a chronic cough developed 2 years ago – extensively investigated but HM has yet to receive a diagnosis

▸ Right ankle fracture – open reduction internal fixation of the right ankle.

Drug history

Drug	Class	Dose	Frequency	Indication
Norethisterone	Progestogen	5 mg	td	Menorrhagia
Tranexamic acid	Antifibrinolytic	1 g	td	Menorrhagia
Co-codamol	Paracetamol + codeine phosphate	30/500 mg	prn	Pain

Allergies

▸ NKDA.

Family history

▸ HM has not spoken to her parents in over 20 years as relations broke down

▸ She has a sister who is well

▸ She says that her father's family has a history of cancer.

Social history

▸ HM lives with her two youngest daughters in a 3-bedroom flat

▸ She is single at the moment; she has seven children to five different fathers, none of whom are in contact with their children

▸ She has had two violent relationships in the past

▸ She previously worked as a cleaner but had to give up due to her respiratory symptoms

- ▸ She is an ex-smoker; she quit 13 years ago
- ▸ She drinks alcohol 'very occasionally'.

Systemic enquiry

- ▸ **Neurological:** Occasional headaches. No faints, fits or dizzy turns. No LOC.
- ▸ **Cardiovascular:** No chest pain.
- ▸ **Respiratory:** SOB, chronic non-productive cough.
- ▸ **Genitourinary:** Constant incontinence. Urgency. Haematuria. No pain.
- ▸ **Gastrointestinal:** No melaena. Generalised abdominal pain. Nausea. Poor appetite.
- ▸ **Musculoskeletal:** Pain and swelling in the right lower leg.

Examination

General

- ▸ HM appears slightly unkempt and is lying comfortably in bed. She is a friendly lady and we established good rapport. There is a distinct smell of necrotic tissue in the room.

Vital signs

- ▸ Temp 36.7°C
- ▸ HR 91 bpm, regular
- ▸ BP 131/72 mmHg.
- ▸ RR 16 breaths/minute
- ▸ BMI 32

Gastrointestinal/abdominal

- ▸ The abdomen is distended in keeping with abdominal obesity
- ▸ Soft and non-tender
- ▸ Active bowel sounds.

Speculum

- ▸ Malignant-looking friable lesion on cervix.

☰ **Summary of patient's problems**

▸ Abdominal pain

▸ Haematuria

▸ Intermenstrual PV bleeding.

❷ **Questions**

▸ Based on the patient's symptoms, what are the main differential diagnoses?

▸ What initial investigations would help confirm the diagnosis?

▸ What is your immediate management plan?

Differential diagnosis

Intermenstrual bleeding:

▶ Hormonal imbalance

> ❯ perimenopausal period: bleeding in this group should be investigated to exclude underlying endometrial cancer

> ❯ breakthrough bleeding due to progesterone-only contraceptive pills

> ❯ breakthrough bleeding due to low-dose oestrogen – too low a prescription, concurrent antiepileptic treatment or diarrhoea

> ❯ contraceptive injection, e.g. Depo-Provera

> ❯ intrauterine contraceptive device

> ❯ anovulatory uterine bleeding

▶ Non-hormonal

> ❯ an ectropion (bleeds spontaneously or after intercourse)

> ❯ cervical polyps or cancer

> ❯ submucosal or pedunculated fibroids (irregular or heavy bleeding)

> ❯ endometrial polyps or cancer

> ❯ inflammatory endometrium due to intrauterine device – a malpositioned device (low lying or abnormally rotated in the uterine cavity) has a higher risk of irregular bleeding and pain

> ❯ infection

>> » endometritis (chlamydia)

>> » gonorrhoea – (less common than chlamydia)

> ❯ drugs which alter clotting – antipsychotics, corticosteroids and anticoagulants

> ❯ pregnancy-related, e.g. ectopic pregnancy.

Management plan

▶ Assess ABCDE

▶ IV access and bloods (FBC, U+Es, LFTs, TFTs, CRP, CA-125)

▶ Analgesia

▶ Antiemetic

▶ IV fluids

▶ CT abdo/pelvis.

Results of investigations

Blood results

▶ Raised WCC and CRP

▶ Acute kidney injury.

CT abdo/pelvis

▶ Bulky cervix and uterus and a collection of cysts in the right ovary.

Diagnosis

▶ Cervical carcinoma

HM is a 48-year-old ex-smoker who presents with a 4-month history of left lower abdominal pain and a 6-week history of heavy intermenstrual PV bleeding. Speculum examination was indicative of cervical malignancy.

Further management plan

▶ Discuss with patient the impact of the diagnosis and offer support

▶ MRI – stage cancer

▶ Gynaecological oncology referral

▶ Discuss at MDT.

Background information: cervical intraepithelial neoplasia and screening

In the UK there are approximately 2800 new cases of cervical cancer each year and 1000 women still die from the disease despite a well-established cervical screening programme. The majority of cases occur in women who have never had a smear, or who have not been regular participants in the screening programme.

Cervical screening

The aim of the cervical screening programme is to detect the non-invasive precursor of the disease known as cervical intraepithelial neoplasia (CIN) in asymptomatic individuals in an attempt to reduce mortality and morbidity. CIN is widely regarded as the precursor lesion for cervical carcinoma and it is a histological diagnosis. Persistent cervical infection with human papillomavirus (HPV) is required for CIN to develop.

The NHS Cervical Screening Programme has been established since 1988. Population screening has been shown to reduce the incidence of cervical cancer and reduce the proportion of women with advanced disease, so the WHO criteria for a screening programme are met. It is thought that the UK screening programme saves 5000 lives per year in the UK.

Since the screening programme began, there has been a 50% reduction in mortality from cervical cancer, and regular cervical screening reduces the risk of death from cervical carcinoma by 75%.

WHO: Wilson–Jungner criteria for appraising the validity of a screening programme

1. The condition being screened for should be an important health problem
2. The natural history of the condition should be well understood
3. There should be a detectable early stage
4. Treatment at an early stage should be of more benefit than at a later stage
5. A suitable test should be devised for the early stage
6. The test should be acceptable
7. Intervals for repeating the test should be determined
8. Adequate health service provision should be made for the extra clinical workload resulting from screening
9. The risks, both physical and psychological, should be less than the benefits
10. The costs should be balanced against the benefits

Screening is based on the natural course of cervical cancer where dysplasia (CIN) precedes the disease. Screening is by cytology of cells taken from the squamocolumnar junction. NICE now recommends liquid-based cytology. All women who are sexually active between the ages of 25 and 64 should be screened. Screening is every 3 years for women aged 25–50 and, if their results are normal, every 5 years until 64 years old.

If the cytology report shows mild dyskaryosis or worse, or if the woman has had two mildly dyskaryotic smears within 6 months, then referral for colposcopy is advised.

Histology of CIN

CIN is characterised by loss of differentiation and maturation from the basal layer of the squamous epithelium upwards.

CIN I	Basal 1/3 of epithelium demonstrates atypia
CIN II	Basal 2/3 of epithelium demonstrates atypia
CIN III	Full thickness

Management of CIN

The management of CIN depends on the grade and patient preference but large loop excision of the transformation zone (LLETZ) is the preferred treatment modality.

Low-grade CIN (CIN I)	Will spontaneously regress in at least 50–60% within 2 years.
	Malignant potential very low but still 10 × greater than normal cytology.
	Management options:
	▸ Conservative monitoring – colposcopy and cytology 6 monthly.
	▸ LLETZ
High-grade CIN (>CIN I)	Will progress to cancer within 10 years in:
	▸ 3–5% – CIN II
	▸ 20–30% – CIN III
	Definitive treatment with LLETZ is necessary.

Background information: cervical carcinoma

Cervical cancer is the second most common malignancy in women worldwide after breast cancer. The mean age at diagnosis is 52 years, but there are two peaks, at 35–39 and 60–64.

Aetiology

The overwhelming majority of cases of cervical cancer are associated with persistent infection with HPV subtypes (mainly 16 and 18). The natural history of the disease has been extensively studied and is well known. As shown in the table on the left, untreated high-grade CIN leads to cervical cancer in 20–30% of women over 10 years.

Risk factors for cervical cancer are:

▸ exposure to HPV:

> early first sexual experience

> multiple partners

> non-barrier contraception (the combined oral contraceptive and high parity may have direct hormonal effects, but it is difficult to show an independent role from indirect effect on sexual behaviour)

▸ smoking: strong dose/response effect – reduced viral clearance

▸ immunosuppression: HIV and transplant patients especially.

Presentation

Approximately 80% of patients are symptomatic. The most common symptom is abnormal vaginal bleeding, e.g. post-coital, intermenstrual or post-menopausal. Rarer presentations, which often suggest advanced disease, include:

▸ heavy PV bleeding

▸ ureteric obstruction

▸ weight loss

▸ bowel disturbance

▸ fistula (vesicovaginal most common).

Investigations

▸ FBC, U+Es, LFTs

▸ CXR – staging and pre-op assessment

▸ MRI – staging

▸ Histology – punch biopsy or small loop biopsy at colposcopy.

FIGO staging of cervical cancer

Stage 0:			Carcinoma *in situ*, intraepithelial carcinoma; cases of stage 0 should not be included in any therapeutic statistics for invasive carcinoma
Stage I:			The carcinoma is strictly confined to the cervix uteri (extension to the corpus should be disregarded)
	IA		Invasive carcinoma that can be diagnosed only by microscopy, with maximum depth of invasion <5 mm
		IA1	Measured stromal invasion <3 mm in depth
		IA2	Measured stromal invasion ≥3 mm and <5 mm in depth
	IB		Invasive carcinoma with measured deepest invasion ≥5 mm (greater than stage IA), lesion limited to the cervix uteri
		IB1	Invasive carcinoma ≥5 mm depth of stromal invasion and <2 cm in greatest dimension
		IB2	Invasive carcinoma >2 cm and <4 cm in greatest dimension
		IB3	Invasive carcinoma ≥4 cm in greatest dimension
Stage II:			The carcinoma invades beyond the uterus, but has not extended onto the lower third of the vagina or to the pelvic wall
	IIA		Involvement limited to the upper two-thirds of the vagina without parametrial involvement
		IIA1	Invasive carcinoma <4 cm in greatest dimension
		IIA2	Invasive carcinoma ≥4 cm in greatest dimension
	IIB		With parametrial involvement but not up to the pelvic wall
Stage III:			The carcinoma involves the lower third of the vagina and/or extends to the pelvic wall and/or causes hydronephrosis or non-functioning kidney and/or involves pelvic and/or paraaortic lymph nodes
	IIIA		Carcinoma involves the lower third of the vagina, with no extension to the pelvic wall
	IIIB		Extension to the pelvic wall and/or hydronephrosis or non-functioning kidney (unless known to be due to another cause)
	IIIC		Involvement of pelvic and/or paraaortic lymph nodes, irrespective of tumour size and extent (with r and p notations)
		IIIC1	Pelvic lymph node metastasis only
		IIIC2	Paraaortic lymph node metastasis

(continued overleaf)

Stage IV:			The carcinoma has extended beyond the true pelvis or has involved (biopsy proven) the mucosa of the bladder or rectum. A bullous oedema, as such, does not permit a case to be allotted to stage IV
		IVA	Spread of the growth to adjacent organs
		IVB	Spread to distant organs

Adapted from Bhatla *et al.* (2019).

Prognosis

Extent of disease	5-year survival
IA	>95%
IB1	90%
IB2	80–85%
II	75–78%
III	47–50%
IV	20–30%

Treatment options

Stage IA1	Local excision plus total abdominal hysterectomy (risk of +ve lymph nodes <1%)
Stage IA2–IB1	Lymphadenectomy + Wertheim's hysterectomy if –ve lymph nodes (Wertheim's hysterectomy involves block dissection of the pelvic lymph nodes and excision of the uterus, tubes, ovaries and upper third of the vagina)
Stage IB2 and early IIA	Radiotherapy Consider lymphadenectomy and Wertheim's hysterectomy in very selected lymph node-negative cases
> Stage IB2	Radiotherapy

Background information: HPV vaccination

All girls can get the HPV vaccine free from the NHS from the age of 12 up to their 18th birthday. The two doses are normally offered 6 to 12 months apart in school year 8 or year 9.

The HPV vaccine is effective at preventing infection by the types of HPV that cause most cervical cancers. Both doses are necessary to be protected.

Resources

Bhatla N, Bherek JS, Cuello Fredes M, *et al.*, Revised FIGO staging for carcinoma of the cervix uteri. *Int J Gynaecol Obstet.* 2019;145:129.

Cancer Research UK. Cervical cancer statistics: www.cancerresearchuk.org/health-professional/cancer-statistics/statistics-by-cancer-type/cervical-cancer

NICE *Guidance on cervical cancer*: www.nice.org.uk/guidance/conditions-and-diseases/cancer/cervical-cancer

Case 23: Prolonged paediatric jaundice

👤 Presenting complaint

▶ LC is a 10-week-old breastfed baby boy who presented with prolonged jaundice.

History of presenting complaint

▶ LC was jaundiced since birth. His bilirubin levels were felt to be within acceptable levels and he did not require phototherapy.

▶ He was discharged after three days.

▶ At his 6-week check, he was still clinically jaundiced, but his bilirubin levels were still thought to be acceptable.

▶ He went for his first immunisations on Wednesday, and the GP recognised his prolonged jaundice and subsequently referred.

▶ His mother feels that the jaundice is visibly improving and says that he is eating and drinking well.

▶ The urine is light yellow in colour and the stools are yellow/green. There has been no change in these since birth. His mother says that he is sleeping most of the night and that he is active when awake. She hasn't noticed any abnormalities in movement or tone.

Past health history

Prenatal history

▶ LC's mother is para 2+0. LC has an older brother who is five and a half years old.

▶ He was born at 40 weeks plus 3 days. There were no complications during the pregnancy including abnormal bleeding, infection or illness.

▶ His mother did not take any medications during her pregnancy.

Birth history

▶ LC weighed 8 lb 6 oz (3.79 kg) and the labour lasted 1.5 hours.

▶ There was no maternal fever or premature rupture of the membranes. It was a vaginal delivery and no intervention was required.

Neonatal period

▶ There was no cyanosis or respiratory distress.

▶ He received vitamin K.

Child development

▸ His mum says that he is very alert and will startle to noises and will fix and follow objects. He will also smile.

▸ His weight is in the 25th percentile.

Immunisations

▸ Up-to-date.

Past medical history

▸ There have been no infections or other illness.

Drug history

▸ Nil.

Allergies

▸ NKDA.

Family history

▸ LC's mother is 36 and his father is 38.

▸ There is no known significant family history including haematological diseases.

Social history

▸ LC lives with his mother, father and older brother in a 3-bed semi-detached house

▸ His mother works as a court clerk but is currently on maternity leave; his father is a kitchen fitter.

Systemic enquiry

Neurological

▸ No history of faints, fits, or 'funny turns'

▸ No febrile seizures

▸ No involuntary movements or tremors.

Respiratory

▸ No history of cough, wheeze or haemoptysis.

Gastrointestinal/abdominal

▶ His appetite is good; he is breastfed every 3 hours

▶ No change in bowel habit (green/yellow-coloured stool).

Physical examination

General

▶ LC is clearly jaundiced. It is most noticeable in his sclera. However, he is alert, smiling and fixing and following on objects. There are no obvious abnormal movements.

Vital signs

▶ Temp 37.2°C

▶ O_2 sats 100% on air

▶ HR: 129 bpm

▶ Weight: 5.2 kg

▶ RR: 38 breaths/minute

Cardiovascular

▶ S1, S2; no added sounds

▶ Peripheral pulses present

▶ No oedema.

Respiratory

▶ No peripheral or central cyanosis

▶ No use of accessory muscles, tracheal tug, or subcostal or intercostal recession

▶ On auscultation, there was no expiratory grunt or inspiratory stridor

▶ There was good air entry throughout.

Gastrointestinal/abdominal

▶ Abdomen was soft and non-tender

▶ Bowel sounds active

▶ No organomegaly and the kidneys were not palpable.

> ### ≔ Summary of patient's problems
> ▶ Prolonged jaundice.

> ### ❷ Questions
> ▶ What are the main differential diagnoses of prolonged jaundice?
> ▶ What initial investigations would help confirm the diagnosis?
> ▶ What is your immediate management plan?

Differential diagnosis

Prolonged jaundice in infants:

▶ Physiological jaundice

▶ Non-physiological unconjugated jaundice

▶ Conjugated jaundice.

Management plan

▶ FBC; blood film; reticulocyte count; clotting ▶ U+E, SBR (total and conjugated), LFT, TFT

▶ Metabolic screen ▶ Group and Coombs

▶ Clear catch urine × 2.

Results of investigations

Blood results

▶ Blood group B +ve ▶ Direct Coombs −ve.

Substance	Reference range	Result
Na⁺	135–145 mmol/L	138 mmol/L
K⁺	3.5–5.0 mmol/L	4.9 mmol/L
Urea	2.5–6.7 mmol/L	2.3 mmol/L
Creatinine	70–150 µmol/L	18 µmol/L
Bilirubin	3–17 µmol/L	153 µmol/L
Conjugated bilirubin		7
ALT	3–35 U/L	25 U/L
AST	3–35 U/L	34 U/L
Alk phos	40–150 U/L	270 U/L
Hb	130–180 g/L	107 g/L
WCC	4–11 × 10⁹/L	8.4 × 10⁹/L
Total protein		60 g/L
Albumin	39–51 g/L	40 g/L

Revised management plan

▶ Seek senior help

▶ Investigate for metabolic disease, e.g. galactosaemia

▶ Abdominal ultrasound

Diagnosis

▶ Prolonged jaundice, ?cause

LC is a 10-week-old breastfed baby boy who presented with prolonged jaundice.

Background information: neonatal jaundice

Neonatal jaundice is one of the most common conditions needing medical attention in newborn babies. About 60% of term and 80% of preterm babies develop jaundice in the first week of life, and about 10% of breastfed babies are still jaundiced at age 1 month.

Jaundice is therefore common, and although it is generally harmless, significant jaundice may indicate serious disease. High serum unconjugated free bilirubin is neurotoxic and can cause deafness, kernicterus (encephalopathy due to deposition of unconjugated bilirubin in the basal ganglia) or athetoid cerebral palsy.

Jaundice can also be a sign of serious liver disease, such as biliary atresia, the prognosis for which is better if it is treated before age 6 weeks. Early recognition of jaundice is therefore vital.

▸ Jaundice occurs when serum bilirubin >25–30 μmol/L.

▸ It is rare outside the neonatal period.

▸ When a baby has jaundice it is important to first determine the serum bilirubin level (SBR) and conjugated (direct) fraction.

▸ Unconjugated jaundice is rarely due to liver disease.

▸ Conjugated jaundice (25 μmol/L) is due to liver disease and requires investigation.

Types of jaundice

Unconjugated jaundice

This is due to excess bilirubin production or impaired liver uptake or conjugation. The causes are:

▸ haemolysis (spherocytosis, G6PD deficiency, sickle-cell anaemia, thalassaemia, haemolytic uraemic syndrome)

▸ Gilbert's syndrome – an autosomal recessive disorder causing underactivity of the conjugating enzyme system bilirubin–uridine diphosphate glucuronyl transferase

▸ Crigler–Najjar syndrome – rare autosomal recessive disorder of bilirubin metabolism.

Intrahepatic cholestasis

This is jaundice due to hepatocyte damage +/– cholestasis. There will be unconjugated +/– conjugated hyperbilirubinaemia. The causes are:

▸ viral hepatitis

▸ drugs – paracetamol overdose, sodium valproate, anti-TB drugs, cytotoxic drugs

▸ Budd–Chiari syndrome

▸ Wilson's disease

▸ Biliary hypoplasia

▸ Alpha-1-antitrypsin deficiency

▸ Hypothyroidism.

Cholestatic (obstructive) jaundice

Conjugated hyperbilirubinaemia due to bile tract obstruction. The causes are:

▸ biliary atresia

▸ choledochal cyst – congenital anomaly of the bile ducts

▸ Caroli's disease – congenital disorder characterised by multifocal, segmental dilatation of large intrahepatic bile ducts

▸ sclerosing cholangitis secondary to IBD

▸ cholelithiasis secondary to chronic haemolysis

▸ cholecystitis

▸ cystic fibrosis

▸ obstructive tumours or cysts.

Neonatal jaundice

Over 60% of all newborn infants become visibly jaundiced. This is because:

▶ there is a marked physiological release of Hb from the breakdown of red cells because of the high Hb concentration at birth

▶ red cells have a shorter lifespan in neonates (70 days vs. 120 days)

▶ hepatic bilirubin metabolism is less efficient in the first few days of life.

Neonatal jaundice is important as:

▶ it may be a sign of another disorder, e.g. haemolytic anaemia, infection, metabolic disease, etc.

▶ unconjugated can lead to kernicterus.

The age of onset is a useful guide to the likely cause of jaundice.

Physiological jaundice

▶ This is common and appears after 24 hours and resolves by 14 days.

▶ It is due to immaturity of hepatic bilirubin conjugation.

▶ Action is only required when SBR is above safe gestation-corrected level (term >260 µmol/L). This should be suspected when jaundice is evident below the umbilicus (jaundice progresses in a cephalic–caudal direction).

Causes of elevated SBR are exaggerated physiological jaundice (e.g. preterm, bruising); sepsis; haemolytic disorders; hepatic disease.

Jaundice in first 24 hours

Jaundice starting within 24 hours of birth usually results from haemolysis (e.g. rhesus haemolytic disease). Other causes include red cell enzyme defects (G6PD deficiency), red cell membrane defects (congenital spherocytosis, elliptocytosis), sepsis, severe bruising.

Prolonged jaundice

Jaundice in babies more than 3 weeks. In most infants the bilirubin will still be unconjugated, but this needs to be confirmed.

In prolonged unconjugated hyperbilirubinaemia:

▶ Breast-milk jaundice is the most common cause (15% of breastfed infants). Usually benign and resolves by 12 weeks.

▶ Infection, particularly UTI, needs to be considered.

▶ Congenital hypothyroidism needs to be excluded.

Conjugated jaundice (SBR >25 µmol/L)

Conjugated hyperbilirubinaemia is suggested by the baby passing dark urine and pale stools.

NICE guidelines on neonatal jaundice

NICE guidelines (CG98, 2016), for all babies:

▶ Check if babies have the following risk factors for developing significant hyperbilirubinaemia:

> visible jaundice in the first 24 hours of life

> a gestational age of <38 weeks

> a previous sibling who had neonatal jaundice needing phototherapy, and/or

> a mother who intends to breastfeed exclusively.

▶ Ensure babies with risk factors for significant hyperbilirubinaemia receive an additional visual inspection by a healthcare professional during the first 48 hours of life.

▶ Examine all babies for jaundice at every opportunity, especially in the first 72 hours. When inspecting for jaundice:

> check the naked baby in bright and preferably natural light

> examine the sclerae, gums and blanched skin in babies of all skin tones.

Babies with jaundice

Measure bilirubin concentrations in all babies with jaundice – do not rely on visual inspection alone to estimate the bilirubin concentration. When measuring the bilirubin concentration:

▸ use a transcutaneous bilirubinometer (a non-invasive device applied to the baby's forehead to measure bilirubin concentrations) in babies with a gestational age of 35 weeks or more and postnatal age of more than 24 hours

▸ if a transcutaneous bilirubinometer is not available, measure the SBR

▸ if a transcutaneous bilirubinometer measurement indicates a bilirubin concentration >250 μmol/L, check the result by measuring the SBR concentration

▸ always use a SBR measurement to determine the bilirubin concentration in (a) babies with jaundice in the first 24 hours of life; (b) preterm babies less than 35 weeks' gestational age; and (c) babies receiving phototherapy.

Management

Use bilirubin concentration to determine management.

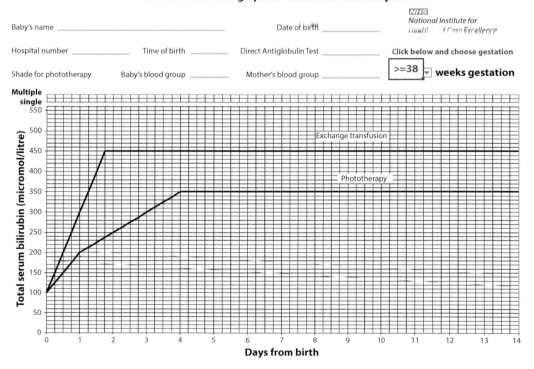

Treatment threshold graph for babies with neonatal jaundice

185

During phototherapy

▶ Using clinical judgment, encourage short breaks for breastfeeding, nappy changing and cuddles unless bilirubin concentrations are approaching the exchange threshold or are rising by more than 8.5 µmol/L per hour.

▶ Continue lactation and feeding support.

▶ Do not routinely give additional fluids or feeds.

▶ Maternal expressed milk is the additional feed of choice if available and when additional feeds are indicated.

Prolonged jaundice

▶ Look for pale, chalky stools and/or dark urine that stains the nappy.

▶ Measure the conjugated bilirubin – raised concentrations may indicate liver disease.

▶ Do a full blood count.

▶ Determine the blood group of the mother and the baby and do a direct antigen test (in the baby); interpret the result and likelihood of Rh disease or other haemolytic disease, taking account of the strength of reaction and whether mother received prophylactic anti-D immunoglobulin during pregnancy.

▶ Arrange a urine culture.

▶ Ensure that routine metabolic screening (including screening for congenital hypothyroidism) has been done.

Follow expert advice for babies with a conjugated bilirubin concentration of >25 µmol/L because this level may indicate serious liver disease.

Resources

NICE *Jaundice in newborn babies under 28 days: CG98* (2016): www.nice.org.uk/guidance/CG98

Chapter 4:

Psychiatry

Case 24: Mania

Presenting complaint

▸ NP is a 57-year-old lady of Pakistani origin who was admitted to the ward at the request of her family. Her family contacted their GP because she had not slept in over a week since she returned from holiday in Pakistan.

History of presenting complaint

▸ NP went to Pakistan on holiday with her husband and son. They had planned to stay there for 3 months, but after a week her family became concerned by her behaviour and had noticed that she wasn't sleeping at night.

▸ She says that when she arrived in Pakistan, Allah started to speak to her. She said that Allah would make comments about her family – 'he's good, he's bad'.

▸ This voice originated from inside her head, and when asked why she was in hospital she replied 'because my husband is a thief and a liar'. NP strongly believes that her husband has another wife and family in Pakistan and says that Allah told her to stab her husband. She doesn't believe that her husband is a bad man but she says that she would still kill him because Allah is all-powerful.

▸ NP also thinks that her husband has a girlfriend named 'Margaret Elizabeth'. NP's son said that there is no evidence of infidelity of any kind.

▸ NP has also experienced visual hallucinations of Allah but she wouldn't elaborate on his appearance or what she sees.

▸ She also has delusions of reference. During our conversation, NP was very restless. She got up from where she was sitting on the bed and went to her wardrobe and produced a magazine telling me that one of the stories was about her. When questioned further, she showed me an article about a man who had killed his two sons and she believed that it involved her.

▸ NP's son says that his mother's behaviour in Pakistan was out of the ordinary. She was 'always on the go' and wasn't sleeping at night. Her appetite remained the same. After a week in Pakistan, she began to make derogatory comments about her husband and would uncharacteristically share her thoughts about him with her family. She also telephoned many members of her family late at night to tell them about her husband's infidelity and her wish to leave him.

▸ She described her mood as high whilst in Pakistan.

▸ She had no thought broadcasting, withdrawal or insertion, and had no suicidal ideation.

▸ She was admitted to a psychiatric hospital in Pakistan for three days but her family were unhappy with the level of care she was receiving and they brought her back to the UK.

Past psychiatric and medical history

▸ Psychiatric admission to hospital in 1972 due to a depressive episode that followed her newborn baby's death at the age of 8 days

▸ Electroconvulsive therapy (ECT) in 1972/73

▸ Essential hypertension

▸ Carpal tunnel syndrome

▸ Diaphragmatic hernia

▸ Reflux oesophagitis

▸ Rheumatoid arthritis

▸ Type 2 diabetes mellitus.

Drug history

Drug	Class	Dose	Frequency	Indication
Mixtard	Biphasic insulin	24 units	bd (8 am, 6 pm)	Diabetes mellitus
Nabumetone	NSAID	500 mg	od	Pain and inflammation in rheumatoid arthritis
Tramadol	Opioid analgesic	50 mg	tds	Pain
Ramipril	ACE inhibitor	10 mg	od	Hypertension
Aspirin	COX inhibitor	75 mg	od	Cardioprotection
Simvastatin	Statin	40 mg	od	Hyperlipidaemia
Metformin	Biguanide	850 mg	od	Diabetes mellitus
Omeprazole	PPI	20 mg	od	Peptic ulcer prophylaxis
Folic acid	Vitamin	5 mg	od	Dually prescribed with methotrexate
Movicol	Osmotic laxative	1 sachet	od	Constipation
Diazepam	Benzodiazepine	5–10 mg	prn	Agitation
Quetiapine XL	Atypical antipsychotic (dopamine antagonist)	400 mg	bd	Mania
Methotrexate	Folate antagonism (inhibits dihydrofolate reductase)	20 mg	once weekly	Rheumatoid arthritis

▸ NP had a recent intramuscular **steroid injection** for her rheumatoid arthritis.

Allergies

▶ NKDA.

Family history

▶ NP's mother, who she says was very religious, had type 1 diabetes and died in her 70s following a stroke

▶ Her father passed away from 'old age'

▶ She says that she had a very good relationship with both her parents

▶ NP has seven sisters and three brothers, and a strong family history of diabetes

▶ She and her husband have four living children (two boys and two girls); in 1972 NP's 8-day-old baby died, and she lost her 2-year-old daughter in 1985 – it was difficult to establish the causes of death

▶ NP also lost another son at the age of 21 years due to 'heart problems' in 1996

▶ NP is visibly deeply distressed at losing her children; she became very upset at this point and began to cry

▶ After speaking to her younger son, it became clear that NP and her husband were having marital difficulties; before the onset of her illness, she had mentioned to family members that she wanted to leave him and that she was unhappy

▶ She says that her husband has a very high sex drive and he will often wake her up in the middle of the night; she says that he constantly wants her to perform oral sex on him and she finds the frequency of this distressing.

Social history

▶ NP had a normal birth. She was born in Pakistan and had a happy childhood.

▶ She attended primary school and then went to secondary school but left after one year because she didn't enjoy it and found the work difficult.

▶ She left at the age of 13 with no qualifications.

▶ She came to the UK in 1972 when she was 19 years old and opened a grocery shop where she worked with her husband.

▶ She is a very religious Muslim and prays 5 times per day.

▶ NP has no forensic history.

▶ NP has never smoked or drunk alcohol.

Premorbid personality

▶ NP's son says that his mother was 'brilliant' before she became acutely unwell in Pakistan. He says that she is a loving wife and mother.

Examination of mental state

Appearance and behaviour

▶ NP was well-dressed in a brightly coloured sari. She was restless and kept getting up from the bed and walking around her room. She maintained eye contact throughout but her eyes appeared 'heavy' and despite her restlessness she still appeared drowsy. Her actions were slow.

▶ Her behaviour was somewhat disinhibited. She repeatedly lifted her top to reveal a scar that was under her left breast. Her son says this is uncharacteristic.

Speech

▶ Her speech was quiet and slow. It was difficult to follow what she was saying at times, and the answers she gave did not always correspond to the questions asked.

Thought form

▶ No abnormality.

Thought content

▶ Delusions of reference regarding a magazine article and delusions involving her husband having another family.

▶ No suicidal ideation.

▶ No thought broadcasting, withdrawal or insertion.

▶ Thoughts of harm towards her husband. She says that it is not her will, but that she is under the control of Allah (? delusions of control).

Mood

▶ Her mood appeared normal. However, there were times when she broke down when discussing her deceased children. She did not seem depressed but was very sad.

Depersonalisation and derealisation thinking

▶ No depersonalisation or derealisation.

Perception

▶ Auditory hallucinations involving Allah. She said that she had seen Him too, but she would not elaborate.

Cognitive function

▶ No abnormality of memory. Concentration was impaired.

Insight

▶ She has no insight into why she was in hospital.

☰ Summary of patient's problems

▶ Recent steroid injection

▶ Insomnia

▶ Disinhibited behaviour

▶ Auditory hallucinations

▶ Delusions.

❓ Questions

▶ Based on the patient's symptoms, what are the main differential diagnoses?

▶ What is your immediate management plan?

Differential diagnosis

▶ Drug-related causes – NP had an intramuscular steroid injection prior to the onset of her symptoms

▶ Mania/manic episode

▶ Hypomania – her episode has been severe enough to warrant hospitalisation and includes psychotic features and so is not hypomania

▶ Bipolar spectrum disorder

▶ Bipolar affective disorder – requires two episodes

▶ Schizophrenia, schizoaffective disorder, delusional disorder, other psychotic disorders

▶ Anxiety disorders/PTSD – no history of anxiety or traumatic events

▶ Circadian rhythm disorders

▶ ADHD

▶ Alcohol or drug misuse – NP is a Muslim and has never smoked or drunk alcohol

▶ Physical illness (e.g. hypo-/hyperthyroidism, Cushing's, SLE, MS, head injury, brain tumour, epilepsy, HIV and other encephalopathies).

Diagnosis

▶ Bipolar affective disorder, current episode manic with psychotic symptoms.

NP is a 57-year-old lady of Pakistani origin who immigrated to the UK in 1972. She has a history of rheumatoid arthritis and received an intramuscular steroid injection prior to her going on holiday to Pakistan. Examination of her mental state revealed disinhibited behaviour and delusional thought content. She had thoughts of harm towards her husband, but no suicidal ideation.

Further management plan

▶ Obtain further history from her family

▶ Bloods (FBC, U+Es, TFT, glucose, LFTs) and full physical examination

▶ Monitor glycaemic control

▶ Urinalysis

▶ Initiate pharmacological treatment – lithium, quetiapine and benzodiazepines. Monitor level of sedation closely due to history of diabetes (i.e. over-sedation vs. hypo).

Background information: bipolar affective disorder

Bipolar affective disorder is characterised by episodes in which the individual's mood is significantly disrupted. The disruption can be as a manic episode in which mood is elevated and energy levels are high, a depressive episode in which mood and energy levels are reduced, or a mixture of the two in which there is marked fluctuation.

To be diagnosed with bipolar affective disorder a patient must have had a manic episode in the past. Any subsequent manic or depressive episodes permit the classification of bipolar affective disorder. This diagnosis is made regardless of whether they have had a depressive episode or not. Subsequent episodes can then be classified as per the ICD-10 classification.

Aetiology

The aetiology of affective disorders is thought to be multifactorial with biological, psychological and social components.

Genetics

Although no region of the genome has been isolated, individuals born to a parent with a bipolar disorder are seven times more to develop the condition and have a 50% chance of developing a psychiatric disorder.

Personality

Cyclothymic personalities (i.e. people prone to mood swings) are at a higher risk of developing a bipolar disorder, though not all will.

Life events

Significant life events can precipitate manic or depressive episodes. These events may be prolonged, like a difficult childhood, or acute, such as a bereavement.

Epidemiology

The lifetime risk of bipolar affective disorder is 0.3–1.5%, with a near-equal distribution between the sexes. The mean age for the first episode is 21.

ICD-10 Classification of bipolar affective disorder	
F31.0	Bipolar affective disorder, current episode hypomanic
F31.1	Bipolar affective disorder, current episode manic without psychotic symptoms
F31.2	Bipolar affective disorder, current episode manic with psychotic symptoms
F31.3	Bipolar affective disorder, current episode mild or moderate depression
F31.4	Bipolar affective disorder, current episode severe depression without psychotic symptoms
F31.5	Bipolar affective disorder, current episode severe depression with psychotic symptoms
F31.6	Bipolar affective disorder, current episode mixed
F31.7	Bipolar affective disorder, currently in remission
F31.8	Other bipolar affective disorders
F31.9	Bipolar affective disorder, unspecified

Clinical features

Clinical features that may be present in manic and depressive episodes

Mania – present for at least 1 week	Depression – present for at least 2 weeks
Elevated mood	Depressed mood
Increased energy and activity	Loss of interest and enjoyment
Decreased sleep	Reduced energy
Pressure of speech	Reduced concentration and attention
Disinhibition	Reduced self-esteem and self-confidence
Poor concentration and attention	Ideas of guilt and unworthiness
Inflated self-esteem	Pessimistic views of the future
Grandiose or over-optimistic ideas	Disturbed sleep
Over-spending	Diminished appetite
Aggression and irritability	Ideas or acts of self-harm or suicide
Flight of ideas	Psychomotor retardation
	Diurnal variation

Episodes may be accompanied by psychotic symptoms such as delusions and hallucinations.

Prognosis

Bipolar disorders are usually cyclical in nature, with recovery between episodes. Each episode usually lasts about 3 months and the first usually occurs before the age of 50. Remission time tends to become shorter as time goes by, and with age the depressive episodes become more common. Poor prognostic factors include poor employment history, alcohol abuse, psychotic features, male sex and non-compliance, while good prognostic factors include later age of onset, few thoughts of suicide and good treatment response and compliance.

Management and treatment

SIGN guidelines (82) for the management of bipolar affective disorder

Acute episodes	
Mania	**Depression**
Antipsychotic drug or semisodium valproate	An antidepressant in combination with an antimanic drug (lithium, semisodium valproate or an antipsychotic drug) or lamotrigine
Lithium: if immediate control of overactive or dangerous behaviour is not needed or otherwise in combination with an antipsychotic	Optimise mood stabiliser drug
Benzodiazepine may be used as an adjunct for sedation	Consider ECT if patient at high risk of suicide or self-harm

(continued overleaf)

Acute episodes	
Mania	**Depression**
Optimise antimanic drug dose – may require combination therapy Treatment-resistant mania may require ECT Reduce and discontinue antidepressant drug treatment	If commencing antidepressant, consider interactions with antipsychotics/lithium and the risk of triggering mania or rapid cycling
Relapse prevention	
Pharmacological	**Psychosocial intervention**
Lithium at an appropriate dose Withdrawal of lithium should be gradual to minimise risk of relapse Carbamazepine as an alternative if lithium ineffective or unacceptable Lamotrigine may be used if initially stabilised on lamotrigine, and if depressive relapse is greater problem	Should be available, especially if complete or continued remission cannot be achieved
Suicide prevention	
Acute and maintenance lithium treatment should be optimised	

Resources

NICE *Bipolar disorder: The management of bipolar disorder in adults, children and adolescents, in primary and secondary care: Clinical guideline 38* (2006): www.nice.org.uk/Guidance/CG38

Case 25: Post-partum psychosis

👤 Presenting complaint

▶ AB is a 22-year-old woman who was admitted as an emergency to the mother-and-baby unit following assessment by the perinatal team. She is 6 weeks post-partum and presented with depressive symptoms, agitation and paranoid ideas.

History of presenting complaint

▶ AB had been having difficulties with her partner of 2 years since the birth of their son.

▶ AB describes a very stressful time since the birth of her son. She was elated after he was born and was looking forward to getting home and looking after him with her partner.

▶ However, she says that her partner, who is in his 40s, was depressed and was reluctant to get involved with the baby. He showed no interest in the baby and said to AB that he was unsure of how he felt towards their child. This resulted in friction between the couple and they had numerous separations over a 6-week period. She felt that she had no stability. This resulted in her moving back to her mother's house with her baby.

▶ She also describes feelings of paranoia and delusional thinking. AB firmly believed that her ex-partner was trying to steal her identity. She also feels that her house was bugged and she taped up the letter box of her mother's house to prevent people getting in. She believed that her ex was spying on her and felt that his friends were watching her house.

▶ She contacted the police to report her concerns but when they arrived she didn't believe that they were real police officers.

▶ She also reported low mood for 2–3 weeks (denies diurnal variation), disturbed sleep with initial insomnia, poor appetite and poor energy levels, lack of enjoyment in life and in spending time with her son, feelings of guilt and worthlessness, feeling ugly and unable to bear to look in the mirror.

▶ She says that for 2–3 days prior to admission, she felt extremely paranoid and was 'jumping from window to window' as she felt she was being watched. She felt hyperactive, didn't sleep and felt obsessive about cleaning.

▶ She used inappropriate language, which was also out of character.

▶ AB describes delusions of reference and said that she felt that television programmes were referring to her and certain songs on the radio triggered memories that were meant only for her.

▶ No thought insertion, withdrawal or broadcasting.

▶ AB describes fleeting feelings of self-harm. However, she didn't make any definitive plans and her baby was a strong protective factor.

▶ She never had any desire to harm her baby.

Past psychiatric and medical history

▸ She had contact with adolescent services in the past due to behavioural disturbance at school and depressive symptoms.

▸ She was discharged due to failure to engage.

▸ No other known psychiatric history.

Medical history

▸ Carpal tunnel syndrome

▸ Gallstones.

Drug history

▸ None.

Allergies

▸ NKDA.

Family history

▸ AB's parents separated when her mother was pregnant with her

▸ When AB was 3 years old her mother met another man and had a son with him

▸ AB first met her biological father when she was 10 years old; her mother and her biological father then got back together briefly – she described this as a difficult time

▸ Her mother is 47 years old and in good health; she is unemployed

▸ She has a good relationship with her mother and feels that they are very close

▸ She has no contact with her biological father

▸ She thinks that her mother and her grandmother both experienced 'depression' in the past but states that it wasn't serious

▸ There is no family history of alcohol or drug abuse.

Social history

▸ She had a normal birth, but her mother was in hospital for a period of 6 months just after the birth due to burns from a deep fat fryer

▸ She had a happy childhood but found her teenage years difficult; she attributes this to the tension between her parents

- She attended two local secondary schools, having to leave her first school because she was on her 'last legs' due to behavioural issues; she 'hated' secondary school and felt that she didn't fit in with the other children her age, and she would always befriend people older than herself

- She left school at 15 with no qualifications, then went to college to study beauty therapy and gained a diploma

- She went on to gain a higher diploma in make-up artistry and gained employment in a department store

- Previous to this she worked with children with special needs, but left this position as it was only temporary

- No forensic history

- AB is a social drinker

- She denies any recreational drugs, but smokes 20 cigarettes/day.

Examination of mental state

Appearance and behaviour

- Well dressed, slightly overweight lady who looks older than her age

- She maintained good eye contact throughout and there was good rapport

- She was feeding her baby during our conversation and she interacted well with him.

Speech

- Normal rate and rhythm.

Thought form

- No abnormality.

Thought content

- Paranoid delusions involving her partner – not as florid as her description during the acute event, but she still describes feelings of paranoia

- No thoughts of self-harm or harm towards her baby at time of assessment.

Mood

- Normal.

Depersonalisation and derealisation

- None.

Perception

- No hallucinations.

Cognitive function

▶ Orientated to time, place and person

▶ No abnormality of immediate recall

▶ Impaired short-term memory

▶ No abnormality of concentration

▶ Average intelligence.

Insight

▶ AB has some insight into her symptoms: she believes what happened with the police to be 'ridiculous' in terms of her not believing they were 'real', and she attributes this to illness

▶ However, she still believes that her delusions involving her husband have some truth and says that she has 'proof'.

≣ Summary of patient's problems

▶ 6 weeks post-partum

▶ Depressive symptoms

▶ Agitation

▶ Paranoid delusions.

---

❷ Questions

▶ Based on the patient's symptoms, what are the main differential diagnoses?

▶ What is your immediate management plan?

Differential diagnosis

▸ Postnatal depression with psychotic symptoms

▸ Post-partum psychosis

▸ Acute stress reaction

▸ Drug-induced state.

Diagnosis

▸ Postnatal depression with psychotic symptoms

AB is a 22-year-old woman who presented 6 weeks post-partum with low mood, biological depressive symptoms and persecutory delusional beliefs. Therefore she was diagnosed with postnatal depression with psychotic features.

Management plan

▸ General observation

▸ Assess risk

▸ Bloods – FBC, U+Es, TFT, LFTs, glucose

▸ Consider toxicology screen

▸ Mid-stream sample of urine

▸ Full physical examination

▸ Consider use of antipsychotic medication.

Background information: post-partum psychosis

Mental disorders during pregnancy and the postnatal period can have serious consequences for the mother, her baby and other family members. The incidence of psychiatric disorders increases greatly after childbirth, with disturbances ranging from mild postnatal blues to severe psychoses.

Maternity blues

This is a transient mood disorder that occurs in up to three-quarters of new mothers 3–5 days after birth. It is well recognised and usually lasts only 2–3 days. Affected mothers may experience tearfulness and emotional lability. Maternal blues usually only requires support and reassurance as the condition is self-limiting.

Postnatal depression

Postnatal depression represents a significant depressive episode that is related to childbirth. It occurs in 10–15% of women within 6 months post-partum, but peaks 3–4 weeks after giving birth. The clinical features include:

▶ tearfulness and profound sadness

▶ poor concentration and indecisiveness

▶ irritability and loss of libido

▶ marked anxiety about the baby's health

▶ negative thoughts of failure and inadequacy as a mother

▶ sleep disturbance

▶ suicidal ideas and thoughts of harm to the baby.

The prognosis is good, with 90% of cases lasting only a month and only 4% lasting longer than one year.

Risk factors for the development of postnatal depression include:

▶ personal or family history of depression

▶ older age

▶ single mother

▶ poor relationship with own mother

▶ poor social support

▶ significant other psychosocial stressors

▶ severe 'baby blues'

▶ previous post-partum psychosis.

These disorders are caused by the psychological adjustments required after childbirth, by loss of sleep and by other factors involved in caring for a new baby.

The management of postnatal depression involves the early identification and monitoring of those at risk. This may be achieved by using such tools as the Edinburgh Postnatal Depression Scale in the primary care setting. Preventative measures include education, antenatal detection, close follow-up and support. Pharmacological treatment of postnatal depression is the same as non-postnatal depression with antidepressants and/or brief cognitive behavioural therapy (CBT). If the symptoms are severe, with suicidal ideation or thoughts of harming the baby, then admission to hospital may be required.

Postnatal psychosis

In almost all cases, postnatal psychosis is a mood disorder accompanied by features such as loss of contact with reality, hallucinations, thought disturbance and abnormal behaviour.

Postnatal psychosis is a much less common condition than postnatal depression and occurs in 1.5/1000 pregnancies. It represents an acute psychotic event that typically is more common in primiparous women and occurs in the first or second week after giving birth. Risk factors for developing postnatal psychosis include:

▶ past history of postnatal psychosis

▶ pre-existing psychiatric disorder

▶ family history of affective disorder in a first- or second-degree relative.

Women who have had a previous postnatal psychosis are at significant risk of future postnatal and non-postnatal episodes. The risk of future postnatal episodes lies between 25% and 57% and the risk of non-postnatal relapse is even higher.

The clinical features of postnatal psychosis closely resemble those of psychoses occurring at other times; however, the women experiencing symptoms of postnatal psychosis are often more deluded, hallucinating, labile and more likely to be disorientated than in non-postnatal psychosis.

As the onset is usually within two weeks after delivery, a biological trigger to the disorder has been proposed. The exact aetiology is unknown, but it is thought that it may relate to a reduction of oestrogen (leading to dopamine super-sensitivity), cortisol levels, or postpartum thyroiditis.

Common clinical features include:

▸ severe insomnia in the absence of a crying baby

▸ confusion and memory impairment

▸ markedly changeable behaviour

▸ paranoid delusions

▸ thought interference

▸ marked guilt, depression, anxiety, irritability

▸ suicidal and/or infanticidal thoughts.

Management

If symptoms are severe, or there are ideas of harm of self or baby, then inpatient treatment is often needed. If the mother is not too disturbed or infanticidal, then admission to a specialist mother-and-baby unit is preferred.

As the nature of postnatal psychosis is essentially affective, treatments used for affective psychoses in general are also appropriate for postnatal psychosis. This includes treatment with:

▸ antipsychotics

▸ antidepressants

▸ ECT for major affective disorder.

Lithium may be used prophylactically to prevent relapse but should not be given to breastfeeding women.

Resources

NICE *Antenatal and postnatal mental health: clinical management and service guidance*, CG192 (2014, updated 2018): www.nice.org.uk/guidance/CG192

Case 26: Schizophrenia

👤 Presenting complaint

HF is a 64-year-old woman with a diagnosis of schizophrenia. She has a long history of psychosis and non-compliance with treatment. She has had multiple psychiatric admissions and was readmitted to hospital at the request of her sister, who was unable to continue caring for her.

History of presenting complaint

▶ HF has been living in a residential setting for many years. However, lately HF's symptoms have become more florid and the carers have found her behaviour difficult to manage.

▶ Recently she has been found wandering at night dressed in inappropriate clothing, she has been disturbing the community priests, and has been pestering local residents by 'visiting' their homes in search of the Archbishop. She is convinced that she can communicate telepathically with the Archbishop.

▶ HF strongly believes that she is a Carmelite nun and says that she wants to go to Lithuania to join a religious order. She continuously picks at her nose as she believes she has stigmata there. She also thinks that she wears a crown of thorns.

▶ She was detained under a short-term detention order and admitted to hospital.

▶ HF's sister was extremely keen to have HF come and live with her and so arrangements were made for this to happen. However, after a week or so, her sister felt that she could no longer care for her and she was readmitted to the psychiatric unit.

Past psychiatric history

▶ HF first presented to psychiatric services at the age of 46 and has remained in contact with services since then

▶ Long-standing problems with schizophrenia that is unfortunately resistant to treatment; she has previously been treated with antipsychotic medication via depot injections

▶ She has refused medication on a number of occasions which results in a deterioration in her symptoms

▶ She describes a number of psychotic experiences including seeing visions of Christ, having stigmata, and tactile hallucinations relating to these.

▶ Previous admissions; increased delusions and refusing food; care staff unable to cope; sister unable to cope.

Medical history

▶ Hypothyroidism, for which she takes thyroxine daily.

Allergies

▸ NKDA.

Family history

▸ HF has a brother and a sister; both parents are deceased

▸ She was married in 1966 and has two daughters and two sons from this relationship, but her husband was abusive and the marriage ended in 1980

▸ She re-married in 1981; she had a son from this relationship before divorcing again in 1985 – her second husband was an alcoholic

▸ She says she has regular contact with her family

▸ No known history of mental illness in the family.

Social history

▸ Her relationship with her mother was often strained – her mother often referred to her as 'ugly' and 'stupid girl'

▸ She had dermatitis as a child and was bullied about this

▸ She attended local schools but found school difficult and did not enjoy it; she left at the age of 15 with no qualifications

▸ HF found employment as a retail assistant and a cleaner, and enjoyed work

▸ She is now retired and receives state benefits

▸ HF was non-compliant with medication and was eventually admitted; this was a lengthy admission

▸ She was placed at a nursing home, but this did not meet her needs and she was placed in residential care

▸ No forensic history

▸ No concerns in relation to drug or alcohol abuse.

Examination of mental state

Appearance and behaviour

▸ Well-dressed

▸ Good eye contact

▸ Repetitive scratching of her nose.

Speech

▸ Normal rate and rhythm.

Thought form

▶ No abnormality.

Thought content

▶ Delusional thought content, as mentioned in the history

▶ She does not have suicidal ideations.

Mood

▶ HF is anxious about her future with regard to joining a religious order in Lithuania.

Depersonalisation and derealisation

▶ None.

Perception

▶ HF experiences tactile hallucinations relating to the stigmata of Christ on her hands, shoulder, forehead and nose

▶ She believes she is telepathically connected to the Archbishop of Glasgow.

Cognitive function

▶ Orientated (time, place, person)

▶ Good attention and concentration

▶ No abnormalities of memory

▶ Average intellect.

Insight

▶ HF has no insight into her current mental health issues and social circumstances.

☰ Summary of patient's problems

▶ Long-standing diagnosis of schizophrenia

▶ Worsening of psychotic symptoms

▶ Hallucinations and delusions.

❓ Questions

▶ What are the main differential diagnoses of psychotic symptoms?

▶ What is your immediate management plan?

Differential diagnosis

Psychotic symptoms:

▸ Schizophrenia

▸ Organic syndromes

In younger patients:

> Drug-induced states (amphetamines and cocaine)

> Temporal lobe epilepsy

In older patients:

> Delirium

> Dementia (finding of a memory disorder suggests dementia)

> Other diffuse brain diseases that can present like schizophrenia, for example, general paralysis of the insane.

▸ Affective disorders (mood disorders with psychotic features)

▸ Anxiety disorders

▸ Personality disorders

▸ Schizoaffective disorders.

Diagnosis

▸ Schizophrenia

HF has a long-standing diagnosis of schizophrenia. Recently her symptoms have become more florid and she was admitted to the psychiatric unit for further management.

Management plan

▸ Admit to the ward and assess risk (risk to themselves, risk of violence towards others)

▸ Investigations: routine bloods – U+Es, LFTs, calcium, FBC, glucose

▸ Consider pharmacological treatment with antipsychotics

▸ Involve HF's sister in long-term management strategy.

Background information: schizophrenia

Schizophrenia is a major psychiatric disorder, or group of disorders, characterised by psychotic symptoms such as delusions and hallucinations, over a spectrum of severity. The patient may experience changes in their thinking and perception and may exhibit a blunted affect and a reduced level of social functioning. Clear consciousness and intellectual capacity are usually spared, although certain cognitive deficits can evolve over the course of the illness.

Clinical features

The symptoms of schizophrenia are ordinarily classified as positive symptoms (an excess or a distortion of normal functioning) and negative symptoms (a decrease or loss of functioning).

- **Positive symptoms** – delusions (commonly persecutory, thought interference, or passivity delusions); hallucinations (usually auditory hallucinations commenting on the subject or referring to them in the third person); formal thought disorder (a loss of the normal flow of thinking, usually shown in the subject's speech or writing).

- **Negative symptoms** – impairment or loss of volition, motivation and spontaneous behaviour; loss of awareness of socially appropriate behaviour and social withdrawal; flattening of mood, blunting of affect and anhedonia; poverty of thought and speech.

Schneider's first-rank symptoms are indicative, though not pathognomonic, of schizophrenia:

- auditory hallucinations: voices discussing the subject in the third person; a running commentary; voices repeating thoughts aloud (thought echo); two or more voices discussing or arguing about the subject

- thought insertion, thought withdrawal, thought broadcasting

- made feelings, actions or somatic passivity (delusions of external control)

- delusional perception.

Diagnosis

The diagnosis of schizophrenia is based entirely on the clinical presentation. Currently, the most widely used diagnostic criteria are those in the ICD-10 and DSM-5. In the DSM-5 classification, symptoms must be present for a minimum of 6 months, whereas in ICD-10, a minimum of 1 month is required to diagnose schizophrenia.

Diagnostic guidelines in the ICD-10 outline the following important psychopathological features for a diagnosis of schizophrenia. Symptoms should include one or more of the following:

- thought echo, insertion, withdrawal or broadcasting

- delusions of control, influence or passivity

- hallucinatory voices

- persistent delusions of other kinds that are culturally inappropriate or implausible.

Or at least two of the following:

- persistent hallucinations in any modality, when accompanied by fleeting or half-formed delusions and over-valued ideas that occur for weeks or months

- breaks in the train of thought, resulting in disorders of thought

- catatonic behaviour

- negative symptoms – apathy, paucity of speech, and blunting or incongruity of emotions.

ICD-10 further categorises schizophrenia into the following types:

- **paranoid schizophrenia** – delusions and hallucinations dominate

- **hebephrenic schizophrenia** – thought disorder and affective disturbance dominate

▸ **catatonic schizophrenia** – catatonia dominates

▸ **undifferentiated** – no specific type dominates

▸ **residual** schizophrenia – negative symptoms dominate.

Epidemiology

The incidence of schizophrenia is similar worldwide. In the UK there are 1–3 new cases per 10 000 population per year. The lifetime risk is approximately 1%, whereas the point prevalence is 0.2–0.7%. The age of onset is between 15 and 40 years, although men tend to have an earlier onset than women (23 years vs. 26 years). Men also tend to develop a more severe illness.

There is an increased prevalence in lower socioeconomic classes (classes IV and V).

The social drift (impairment of functioning caused by schizophrenia results in a 'drift' down the social scale) and social causation (poor socioeconomic conditions contribute to the development of schizophrenia) theories attempt to explain this.

The incidence rate is also higher for immigrants – in the UK, especially Afro-Caribbeans.

Suicide is the most common cause of premature death in schizophrenia. It accounts for 10–38% of all deaths in this group.

Aetiology

The aetiology of schizophrenia is uncertain. However, a number of risk factors are known and it is thought that a complex interaction between the individuals' genetics and their environment are involved.

Risk factors in schizophrenia

	Biological	Psychological	Social
Predisposing factors	Genetic Prenatal factors – abnormalities of pregnancy and birth, maternal influenza, foetal malnutrition, winter birth Heavy cannabis consumption.	Schizotypal personality	Urban environment Under-stimulating environment Low social class
Precipitating factors	Illicit drugs	Stressful life events	Psychosocial stresses
Perpetuating factors	Non-compliance with treatment Drug use	Stressful life events	High expressed emotion
Mediating factors	Neurochemical theories – D1/2/3 + 5HT		

Inheritance

Genetic factors account for the majority of liability to schizophrenia.

Schizophrenia liability based on affected relatives

Family member(s) affected	Risk (approx.)
Identical twin	46%
One sibling/fraternal twin	12–15%
Both parents	40%
One parent	12–15%
One grandparent	6%
No relatives affected	0.5–1%

Other theories exist on the aetiology of schizophrenia.

▸ Dopamine hypothesis – the fact that all known effective antipsychotics are dopamine antagonists suggests that an excess of dopamine is involved.

▸ There are also theories involving serotonin or glutamate neurotransmitter systems.

▸ Neurodevelopmental hypothesis – structurally, brains of people with schizophrenia have enlarged ventricles and reduced cortical grey matter. Functionally, abnormalities are found in the frontal and temporal lobes.

Management

The management of schizophrenia aims to improve symptoms and prevent relapse. A method aimed at tackling the biopsychosocial aspects of schizophrenia is preferred.

Pharmacological therapies

The use of atypical antipsychotics (olanzapine, risperidone) is recommended as first-line treatment for newly diagnosed patients and for patients on typical antipsychotics who experience inadequate symptom control or unacceptable side-effects.

Typical antipsychotics are effective at treating positive symptoms (delusions, hallucinations, disorganised thinking) but may fail to treat negative symptoms (apathy, poverty of thought and speech). They are associated with extrapyramidal side-effects (EPSEs: Parkinson-like symptoms, acute dystonia, akathisia), tardive dyskinesia (24% of patients), neuroleptic malignant syndrome (rare, life-threatening reaction to antipsychotic medication – fever, muscular rigidity, altered mental status, autonomic dysfunction) and hyperprolactinaemia. Parkinsonism and acute dystonias should be promptly treated with anticholinergics (e.g. procyclidine).

Atypical antipsychotics are at least as effective as the typical antipsychotics in

Biological	Psychological	Social
Pharmacological treatment: ▸ antipsychotics ▸ benzodiazepines ▸ lithium ▸ antidepressants ▸ anticholinergic drugs for EPSEs ECT – treat cases of catatonic stupor and severe depressive symptoms	CBT and family psychological interventions may be useful in preventing relapses	Supportive care from community nurses Social skills training Employment training

treating positive symptoms and may improve negative symptoms, mood symptoms, and perhaps cognition as well. They are less likely to cause EPSEs and tardive dyskinesia, and thus lead to improved compliance. Clozapine, quetiapine and, to a lesser extent, olanzapine, are prolactin-sparing. Despite these major benefits, several side-effects have emerged that may limit the utility of some of those medications.

Medication side-effects
Agranulocytosis: clozapine
Diabetes, weight gain, lipid abnormalities: clozapine, olanzapine and quetiapine
Increased prolactin levels (galactorrhoea, sexual dysfunction, osteoporosis): risperidone and amisulpride

Treatment-resistant schizophrenia is defined as a lack of satisfactory clinical improvement despite the sequential use of at least two antipsychotics for 6–8 weeks, one of which should be atypical. In these instances, patients should be started on clozapine at the earliest opportunity. Clozapine is not used as a first-line therapy due to its potential to cause life-threatening agranulocytosis in just less than 1% of patients. Thus, regular haematological monitoring is necessary and patients are required to be registered with a monitoring service. Clozapine will benefit over 60% of treatment-resistant patients.

Resources

NICE *Psychosis and schizophrenia in adults: prevention and management*, CG178 (2014): www.nice.org.uk/ Guidance/CG178

Case 27:   Alcohol detoxification

👤 Presenting complaint

▶ MF was admitted as part of an alcohol detoxification programme. She has been experiencing deep, throbbing pains in her right upper quadrant and lower back for approximately 9 months. She attributes this pain to excess alcohol consumption.

History of presenting complaint

▶ MF has been drinking excessively and using drugs for 32 years. At the age of 17, she started to take non-prescribed diazepam as her boyfriend at the time was experimenting with drugs.

▶ This relationship was extremely damaging and abusive, and MF found herself being manipulated and forced into prostitution. She worked as a prostitute for the next 10 years.

▶ During this time, she started using heroin. Initially, she smoked a £10 bag/day but this quickly escalated over a period of months to her injecting £50–60 bags/day. MF's habit was funded through prostitution.

▶ She stopped using heroin 3 years ago and is now on a methadone programme. She was initially taking 120 mL of methadone per day. At present she is taking 40 mL/day and she is slowly reducing this dose. Her dose is reduced at 5 mL/month.

▶ MF feels that her main problem at this time is her alcohol intake. She has a long history of alcohol abuse and fears that if she is unable to stop drinking then it may kill her.

▶ She wakes up at 8 am, if she has slept at all, and will drink half a bottle of vodka. She says that she has to drink to stop shaking. Her typical day is planned around alcohol and she has been drinking more than 1 L of vodka a day for several months. She describes abdominal swelling and says that it makes her 'look pregnant'.

▶ Her mood is low and she believes that she is depressed and has been for many years. She describes herself as 'weepy' and says that she sleeps excessively during the day and is awake most of the night. She rarely leaves the house.

Past psychiatric and medical history

▶ Numerous past depressive episodes; MF believes she has been depressed since childhood

▶ Two previous suicide attempts: one at the age of 19 when, following the death of her father, an alcoholic, MF reports that she took 60 × 10 mg of diazepam

▶ The second attempt occurred when MF was in her 20s and homeless after her mother threw her out of the family home for prostitution. This was a difficult time for MF and she tried to end her life by taking an undisclosed amount of amitriptyline. It was an impulsive attempt, with no suicide note or preparation. She says that she was not under the influence of any other drugs or alcohol at the time

▸ MF states that she intended to die on both occasions and felt angry at waking up in hospital

▸ She has had multiple psychiatric admissions for depressive symptoms and rehabilitation for heroin and alcohol addiction. MF was also diagnosed with hepatitis C in 1989.

Drug history

Drug	Class	Dose	Frequency	Indication
Chlordiazepoxide	Benzodiazepine	10 mg	tid (for 3 days) bid (2 days)	Alcohol withdrawal
		15 mg	od (one day)	
		10 mg	od (one day)	
Thiamine	Vitamin B1	100 mg	bd	Prophylactic for Wernicke–Korsakoff's
Forceval	Vitamin and mineral supplement	1 cap	daily	Prophylaxis for vitamin deficiency
Quinine	Alkaloid	200 mg	od nocte	Leg cramps
Pabrinex	Vitamin B1	Amps 1+2	od	Prophylaxis for Wernicke–Korsakoff's

Allergies

▸ NKDA.

Family history

▸ MF's mother is 68 years old, has emphysema and angina, and is registered blind

▸ MF's relationship with her mother is strained after her mother threw her out of the house when she was 19 years old – MF resents her mother for this and feels that her mother could have done more to help

▸ Her father passed away at the age of 39 due to years of alcohol abuse

▸ Her memories of her father are very negative: she says that her childhood was difficult due to neglect and her father's drinking – 'we had nothing, but my dad could always afford a drink'

▸ MF has three sisters aged 40, 44 and 47, all of whom are alcoholics, and a brother who does not drink alcohol but does use amphetamines heavily

▸ She has a son who is 28 years old

▸ Her son went to stay with his grandmother at the age of 4 when MF was 20 and will not communicate with MF; she has tried to keep contact but her son does not want to be involved in her life. She showed very little emotion when discussing this topic

- MF lost a child at the age of three days old as a result of spina bifida; the child had a different father than her other son
- There is no family history of serious mental illness but her mother had a 'breakdown' when she was in her 40s.

Social history

- MF's mother had a normal pregnancy and birth
- She had an unhappy childhood which she attributes to her father, who was violent and abusive towards MF's mother; she remembers asking her mother to leave him on a number of occasions
- Financial problems were common throughout her childhood and she had to share a bed with her three sisters
- MF attended three separate primary schools because her family were routinely evicted from their homes as a result of her father not paying the rent or household bills
- She also attended two secondary schools, leaving the first because she moved away to live with her aunt when she could no longer tolerate her father's behaviour
- She left school at 16 with no qualifications and worked in a hotel for 2 years
- She then met her then boyfriend and spent the next 10 years in prostitution
- She now receives state benefits
- MF has been in her current relationship for 21 years, which, she says, can be extremely volatile at times due to alcohol: her partner has never taken drugs and is only a moderate drinker, but she is at times violent towards him and she will often attack him, pulling his hair and scratching him when she is intoxicated
- MF has had multiple short detentions in prison for unpaid fines in relation to prostitution
- She has no outstanding charges.

Examination of mental state

Appearance and behaviour

- Smart and well-dressed lady who was 'doing' her make-up during our conversation
- She appears bloated and had abdominal swelling; she looks older than her age
- Good interaction and eye contact.

Speech

- Normal rate and rhythm
- Articulate.

Thought form

▸ No abnormality.

Thought content

▸ No delusions or suicidal ideation.

Mood

▸ Normal mood.

Depersonalisation and derealisation

▸ None.

Perception

▸ No hallucinations or illusions.

Cognitive function

▸ No problems with immediate recall: when asked to repeat the address '15 Burns Street', she did so

▸ However, short-term memory was impaired. When asked to repeat the same address after 5 minutes her reply was '10 Burns St'

▸ No abnormalities of attention

▸ Concentration impaired

▸ MF had great difficulty with serial 7s, and was unable to subtract 7 from 100.

Insight

▸ MF is very insightful into her current situation and understands that alcohol is a major problem in her life.

≔ Summary of patient's problems

▸ Alcohol and drug dependency
▸ Chaotic lifestyle/prostitution
▸ Low mood.

Diagnosis

▶ Planned admission for alcohol detoxification

MF has long-standing issues surrounding alcohol dependence. She is keen to abstain from alcohol and was admitted for alcohol detoxification.

Management plan

▶ A biopsychosocial approach to managing this patient is needed

▶ Undertake baseline BP, temperature and pulse and then monitor as required (at least 4-hourly) for first 48 hours

▶ Check for hypoglycaemia and/or dehydration on admission and then as necessary

▶ FBC, LFTs, U+Es

▶ Initiate withdrawal regime of chlordiazepoxide for 7 days

▶ Review patient's response at an early stage so that further dose titration can take place where necessary

▶ Supplementary vitamins (parenteral thiamine)

▶ Individual or group counselling

▶ AA and relapse prevention

▶ CBT

▶ Involve the family whenever possible.

Background information: alcohol withdrawal syndromes

When a person is dependent on alcohol, stopping alcohol completely or significantly reducing the usual amount taken can result in the development of characteristic withdrawal syndromes. These syndromes are common in a patient who has:

▶ a history of dependence

▶ previously experienced withdrawal syndromes

▶ consumed more than 10 units of alcohol on a daily basis for the previous 10 days.

The alcohol withdrawal syndromes may be uncomplicated or may involve seizures and delirium tremens.

An **uncomplicated alcohol withdrawal syndrome** usually occurs 4–12 hours after the last alcoholic drink, The features include:

▶ tremor

▶ sweating

▶ insomnia

▶ tachycardia

▶ nausea and vomiting

▶ psychomotor agitation

▶ generalised anxiety

Occasionally there may also be visual, auditory and tactile hallucinations. The individual may crave alcohol in itself and as a relief from the symptoms mentioned above. Symptoms peak 48 hours after cessation of alcohol and last approximately 2–5 days. Symptom severity relates to the amount of alcohol consumed.

In 5–15% of cases withdrawals are complicated by **seizures** which usually occur 6–48 hours after the last drink. Predisposing factors include previous history of withdrawal seizures, epilepsy, history of head injury, and hypokalaemia.

Delirium tremens is the most severe form of alcohol withdrawal and represents a medical emergency that requires inpatient medical care. It is thought to occur in about 5% of cases of alcohol withdrawal. Symptoms manifest 1–7 days after the last alcoholic drink and peak within 2 days. In addition to the symptoms of uncomplicated withdrawal, patients also experience:

▶ clouding of consciousness

▶ disorientation

▶ amnesia of recent events

▶ marked psychomotor agitation

▶ visual, auditory and tactile hallucinations (characteristically of diminutive people or animals – 'Lilliputian hallucinations')

▶ marked fluctuations in the severity of symptoms – usually worse at night

▶ when severe: heavy sweating, fear, paranoid delusions, agitation, raised temperature, sudden cardiovascular collapse.

Delirium tremens is a serious condition and mortality is reported in 5–10% of patients. It is most severe when it is sudden and when it occurs in an individual who is not known to be alcohol dependent.

Management

Alcohol withdrawal may be dangerous and requires careful clinical management. Detoxification, the planned withdrawal of alcohol, involves providing the patient with psychological support, prescribing medication to relieve withdrawal symptoms, observation for the development of features suggestive of complicated withdrawal, nutritional supplementation and an integrated follow-up. The initial problems of withdrawal are short-lived and the major difficulty in managing alcohol dependence is the inability to maintain abstinence.

Detoxification may be an inpatient treatment or carried out in the community. For patients with mild to moderate withdrawal symptoms, it should be possible to safely and effectively detoxify patients in the community as an outpatient over the course of 1 week. This is the treatment of choice for most uncomplicated cases.

Hospital detoxification is advised if the patient:

▶ is confused or has hallucinations

▶ has a history of previously complicated withdrawal

▶ has epilepsy or has fits

▶ is undernourished

▶ has severe vomiting or diarrhoea

▶ has severe dependence coupled with unwillingness to be seen daily

▶ is at risk of suicide

▶ has a previously failed home attempt

▶ has uncontrollable withdrawal symptoms

▶ has multiple substance misuse

▶ has a home environment unsupportive of abstinence.

Medication

Medication is not necessary for treatment of withdrawal if the patient's alcohol consumption is less than 15 units/day in men or 10 units/day in women, and if the patient reports neither recent withdrawal symptoms nor recent drinking to prevent withdrawal symptoms.

Among periodic drinkers whose last bout was less than one week long, medication is seldom necessary unless drinking is extremely heavy (>20 units/day).

When medication to manage withdrawal is not given, patients should be told that at the start of the detoxification they may feel nervous or anxious for several days, with difficulty in going to sleep for several nights.

Medications used in the management of withdrawal are listed below.

Benzodiazepines: Alcohol enhances the inhibitory effects of the neurotransmitter GABA and diminishes the activity of the excitatory NMDA receptors. Pharmacotherapy is therefore based on depressant drugs that enhance GABA.

Benzodiazepines are prescribed in a rapidly reducing regime. Chlordiazepoxide is first-line drug treatment as it is slowly absorbed, has a long half-life and low potency, and therefore low addictive potential.

Benzodiazepine withdrawal regime

	On waking	Midday	Early evening	At bedtime
Day 1	–	30 mg	30 mg	30 mg
Day 2	20 mg	20 mg	20 mg	20 mg
Day 3	20 mg	10 mg	10 mg	10 mg
Day 4	10 mg	10 mg	–	20 mg
Day 5	10 mg	–	–	10 mg

Biological	Psychological	Social
Pharmacological therapy: ▸ disulfiram (Antabuse) ▸ acamprosate (Campral)	Motivational interviewing: moves patients through a cycle: 'precontemplation' → 'contemplation' → 'determination' → 'action' → 'maintenance' CBT: exposure, relapse prevention work, behavioural contracting Group therapy AA	Social support: social workers, probation officers and Citizens Advice agencies may be able to help with homelessness, criminal charges and debt Patients may have to be advised to alter leisure activities or change jobs if these are contributing to the problem

Other medications:

▸ Antipsychotics – haloperidol 5–10 mg orally up to tds for hallucinations and delusions. These may lower the seizure threshold, but benzodiazepines should cover this.

▸ Supplementary vitamins – to prevent Wernicke–Korsakoff syndrome, give parenteral B vitamins.

Maintenance therapy after detoxification:

The treatment of alcohol dependence involves more than just 'detoxification'.

The management of dependence involves addressing all the psychological, biological and sociocultural factors that have led to its development.

Resources

NICE *Alcohol-use disorders: diagnosis, assessment and management of harmful drinking and alcohol dependence, CG115* (2011): www.nice.org.uk/guidance/CG115

Appendix:

Figure acknowledgements

Case 1: Progressive dyspnoea

Chest X-ray – reproduced with permission from: http://learningradiology.com/lectures/cardiaclectures/Congestive%20Heart%20Failure-2012/Congestive%20Heart%20Failure-2012.html

ECG – reproduced from: https://commons.wikimedia.org/wiki/File:Cardiogram_indicating_right_bundle_branch_block.jpg under a Creative Commons Attribution-Share Alike 3.0 Unported licence. Attribution: James Heilman, MD

Case 2: Wheeze

CXR – reproduced from: https://physioknowledgebd.blogspot.com/2016/03/asthma-imaging.html

Case 3: Chest pain

ECG – reproduced from: https://lifeinthefastlane.com/ecg-library/anterior-stemi/

Case 4: Dyspnoea and confusion

COPD staging – reproduced from: www.quora.com/how-clearly-defined-and-meaningful-is-the-diagnosis-of-first-stage-COPD

Case 5: Back pain and breathlessness

CXR – reproduced with permission from: https://cancerdundee.wordpress.com/image-of-the-week/a-cxr/

Case 6: Headache

CT head – reproduced from: http://casemed.case.edu/clerkships/neurology/Web%20Neurorad/mcaanery2a.htm

Case 9: Deteriorating vision

Fundoscopy – reproduced from: https://commons.wikimedia.org/wiki/File:Hypertensiveretinopathy.jpg. Attribution: Frank Wood

Case 10: Abdominal pain

CXR – reproduced from: https://en.wikipedia.org/wiki/Pneumoperitoneum under a Creative Commons Attribution-Share Alike 2.5 Generic Licence. Attribution: Clinical_Cases

Case 12: Acute loin pain and haematuria

CT KUB – reproduced from: https://commons.wikimedia.org/wiki/File:3mmstone.png under a Creative Commons Attribution-Share Alike 3.0 Unported Licence. Attribution: James Heilman, MD

Case 14: Abdominal pain and jaundice

Cullen and Grey Turner signs – reproduced with permission from: www.60secondem.com/visual-diagnosis-16-answers/

Case 16: Haematuria

Tumour node classification reproduced with permission of John Wiley and Sons, from: Union for International Cancer Control, *TNM Classification of Malignant Tumours*, 8th edition (eds J.D. Brierley, M.K. Gospodarowicz and C. Wittekind). © 2017 UICC.

Case 18: Crohn's disease: abdominal pain and vomiting

AXR – reproduced with permission from Medscape Drugs & Diseases (https://emedicine.medscape.com/), Small-Bowel Obstruction Imaging, 2016, available at: https://emedicine.medscape.com/article/374962-overview

Case 23: Prolonged paediatric jaundice

Bilirubin management chart – © NICE 2010 (updated 2016) CG98. Available from www.nice.org.uk/guidance/CG98 All rights reserved. Subject to notice of rights. NICE guidance is prepared for the National Health Service in England. All NICE guidance is subject to regular review and may be updated or withdrawn. NICE accepts no responsibility for the use of its content in this product/publication.